Sleep Issues in Neuromuscular Disorders

Raghav Govindarajan • Pradeep C. Bollu
Editors

Sleep Issues in Neuromuscular Disorders

A Clinical Guide

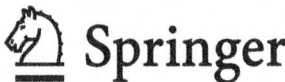

Editors
Raghav Govindarajan
Department of Neurology
University of Missouri
Columbia
Missouri
USA

Pradeep C. Bollu
Department of Neurology
University of Missouri
Columbia
Missouri
USA

ISBN 978-3-030-10309-5   ISBN 978-3-319-73068-4   (eBook)
https://doi.org/10.1007/978-3-319-73068-4

© Springer International Publishing AG, part of Springer Nature 2018
Softcover re-print of the Hardcover 1st edition 2018
This work is subject to copyright. All rights are reserved by the Publisher, whether the whole or part of the material is concerned, specifically the rights of translation, reprinting, reuse of illustrations, recitation, broadcasting, reproduction on microfilms or in any other physical way, and transmission or information storage and retrieval, electronic adaptation, computer software, or by similar or dissimilar methodology now known or hereafter developed.
The use of general descriptive names, registered names, trademarks, service marks, etc. in this publication does not imply, even in the absence of a specific statement, that such names are exempt from the relevant protective laws and regulations and therefore free for general use.
The publisher, the authors and the editors are safe to assume that the advice and information in this book are believed to be true and accurate at the date of publication. Neither the publisher nor the authors or the editors give a warranty, express or implied, with respect to the material contained herein or for any errors or omissions that may have been made. The publisher remains neutral with regard to jurisdictional claims in published maps and institutional affiliations.

Printed on acid-free paper

This Springer imprint is published by the registered company Springer International Publishing AG part of Springer Nature
The registered company address is: Gewerbestrasse 11, 6330 Cham, Switzerland

To,

Our beloved families, colleagues, students, and most importantly our patients who have inspired to complete this work.

Preface

Sleep issues are common in patients with neuromuscular disorders. While neuromuscular physicians are trained in managing complex neuromuscular conditions and have a firm grasp on neurophysiology, pathology, and genetics, sleep and sleep-related issues can be challenging. Similarly sleep specialists have a firm grasp on understanding sleep neurobiology, pathology, and managing sleep issues including neuromuscular respiratory weakness but might find it challenging to understand the ever evolving and diverse field of neuromuscular disorders. With this in mind, we have designed this handbook for both neuromuscular physicians and sleep specialists by providing clinically relevant material in both sleep medicine and neuromuscular medicine that a busy clinician will find useful for a quick reference. Further, the book will be highly beneficial to any practicing physician including pulmonary/critical care physicians, neuro ICU physicians, primary care doctors and internists who take care of neuromuscular patients, pediatricians, general neurologists and even advanced practice providers, fellows, residents, respiratory therapists, and medical students. This guide is meant to help them understand the basics of sleep and neuromuscular disorders and its clinical management but is not a comprehensive review.

This book has been divided into ten chapters. Chapters 1 and 2 lay the foundation for understanding sleep issues in neuromuscular disorders. Chapters 3–7 provide an overview of sleep disorders in various neuromuscular conditions. Finally, Chaps. 8–10 provide practical advice in managing sleep issues including an overview of noninvasive ventilation. The final part of the book provides useful tables, charts, pictures, and flow charts for quick reference in sleep medicine and neuromuscular medicine.

We are very thankful to all our colleagues and coauthors who have spent numerous hours preparing the chapters. In addition, we are grateful to our chairman Dr. Pradeep Sahota for his guidance and mentorship throughout the project. Last but not least, we thank Springer for their input in putting this book together.

Columbia, MO   Pradeep C. Bollu, M.D.
Columbia, MO   Raghav Govindarajan, MD, FAAN, FAMWA,
FISQua, FACSc, FCPP, MAcadMEd, FASA

Contents

1 **The Basics of Polysomnography** 1
Prashanth Natteru and Pradeep C. Bollu

2 **Neuromuscular Respiratory Failure** 23
Miguel Chuquilin and Nakul Katyal

3 **Sleep Issues in Motor Neuron Diseases** 43
Sushma Yerram, Pradeep C. Bollu, and Pradeep Sahota

4 **Sleep Issues in Myopathic Disorders and Muscular Dystrophies** 61
Valentina Joseph, Joe Devasahayam, and Munish Goyal

5 **Sleep Issues in Neuromuscular Junction Disorders** 73
Prashant Natteru, Siva Pesala, Pradeep C. Bollu, and Raghav Govindarajan

6 **Sleep Disorders in Peripheral Neuropathy** 95
Satish Bokka, Raghav Govindarajan, and Nakul Katyal

7 **Sleep Issues in Pediatric Neuromuscular Disorders** 101
Raja Boddepalli and Raghav Govindarajan

8 **Basics and Practical Aspects of Non-invasive Mechanical Ventilation** 117
Joe Devasahayam, Troy Whitacre, and Tony Oliver

9 **Non-invasive Ventilation in NeuroMuscular Diseases** 129
Hariharan Regunath, Troy Whitacre, and Stevan P. Whitt

10 **Trouble Shooting with Noninvasive Ventilation** 139
Vijay Kodadhala and Pradeep C. Bollu

Appendix 153

Index 165

Contributors

Raja Boddepalli, M.D. Academic Department, Stony Brook University School of Medicine, Stony Brook, NY, USA

Satish Bokka, M.D. Department of Neurology, University of Louisville School of Medicine, Louisville, KY, USA

Pradeep C. Bollu, M.D. Department of Neurology, University of Missouri, Columbia, MO, USA

Miguel Chuquilin, M.D. Department of Neurology, University of Florida, Gainesville, FL, USA

Joe Devasahayam, M.D. University of Missouri, Columbia, MO, USA

Raghav Govindarajan, MD, FAAN, FAMWA, FISQua, FACSc, FCPP, MAcadMEd, FASA Department of Neurology, University of Missouri, Columbia, MO, USA

Munish Goyal, M.D. Department of Neurology, University of Missouri, Columbia, MO, USA

Valentina Joseph, M.D. Neurology and Sleep Medicine, University of South Dakota-Sanford School of Medicine, Sioux Falls, SD, USA

Vijay Kodadhala, M.D. Fellow in Pulmonary Medicine, Howard University Hospital, Washington, DC, USA

Prashanth Natteru, M.D. Department of Neurology, University of Mississippi Medical Center, Jackson, MS, USA

Tony Oliver, M.D. Sanford Medical Center, University of South Dakota, Sioux Falls, SD, USA

Siva Pesala, M.D. Department of Neurology, University of Missouri, Columbia, MO, USA

Hariharan Regunath, M.D. Divisions of Pulmonary, Critical Care and Infectious Diseases, Department of Medicine, University of Missouri, Columbia, MO, USA

Pradeep Sahota, M.D., F.A.A.N. Department of Neurology, University of Missouri, Columbia, MO, USA

Troy Whitacre, R.R.T. Respiratory Therapy Services, University of Missouri Hospital and Clinics, Columbia, MO, USA

Stevan P. Whitt, M.D. Division of Pulmonary, Critical Care and Environmental Medicine, Department of Internal Medicine, University of Missouri, Columbia, MO, USA

Sushma Yerram, M.D. Department of Neurology, University of Rochester, Rochester, NY, USA

The Basics of Polysomnography

Prashanth Natteru and Pradeep C. Bollu

Introduction

The word "polysomnography" was derived from Greek and Latin. The word "poly" stands for many; "somnus" for sleep, and finally "graphein" is to write [1].

Polysomnography: The Beginning

In 1874, a Scottish physiologist Richard Caton (1842–1926) first noticed "feeble currents of varying direction" in the brains of rabbits and monkeys and described it as electrical potential changes related to the brain activity [2, 3]. It was not until 1924, when a psychiatrist from Jena, Germany, Johannes (Hans) Berger (1873–1941) recorded the first cortical electrical activity in man. His observation of the alpha rhythm when awake, and its disappearance on falling asleep, finally led to the electroencephalogram (EEG) coming into existence [4]. This discovery opened up new horizons in sleep research: establishing the presence of brain activity during sleep, and the possibility of objectively quantifying it [5].

Nathaniel Kleitman, universally recognized as father of sleep research, was a Professor of Physiology at University of Chicago. In the early 1920s, he set up a laboratory exclusively dedicated to sleep research. He conducted several experimental sleep recordings and was pivotal in the discovery of rapid eye movement (REM) sleep [5]. Eugene Aserinsky, a graduate student of Professor Kleitman at

P. Natteru, M.D.
Department of Neurology, University of Mississippi Medical Center, Jackson, MS, USA
e-mail: pnatteru@umc.edu

P. C. Bollu, M.D. (✉)
Department of Neurology, University of Missouri, Columbia, MO, USA
e-mail: BolluP@health.missouri.edu

© Springer International Publishing AG, part of Springer Nature 2018
R. Govindarajan, P. C. Bollu (eds.), *Sleep Issues in Neuromuscular Disorders*,
https://doi.org/10.1007/978-3-319-73068-4_1

University of Chicago sleep laboratory, was assigned the task of observing people's eye movements in sleep. He used to observe infants in their homes during the day, and adults in the sleep laboratory at night. Observing people's eye movements during sleep at night was a tiresome task, so they innovated an easier way of recording eye movements, by placing electrodes on the skin adjacent to the eyeballs. And just like that, was born the electrooculogram (EOG). In 1953, Aserinsky and Kleitman published a paper describing the "rapid eye movement" (REM) periods on EOG, and its association with a rich dream recall " [6].

William Charles Dement who is considered as the father of modern sleep science worked along with Dr. Kleitman helped identify the different stages of sleep. He was the founder of the Sleep Research Center—the world's first sleep disorders clinical unit at Stanford University, in 1964. He established the American Sleep Disorders Association in 1975, now known as the American Academy of Sleep Medicine (AASM) [5].

In 1959, Michel Valentin Marcel Jouvet, a neurophysiologist conducted several experiments on cats regarding muscle atonia during REM sleep. He demonstrated that an intact pontine tegmentum is imperative for the generation of REM sleep and that an inhibition of motor centers in the medulla oblongata leads to REM atonia. Cats with lesions in the vicinity of locus coeruleus showed less restricted muscle movement during REM sleep, and a diversity of complex behaviors, including motor patterns suggesting that they are dreaming of an attack, defense, and exploration. He also illustrated the absence of muscle potentials during the REM periods in cats. He identified REM sleep as an independent state of alertness and termed it as "paradoxical sleep" [7, 8]. Thereafter, the emphasis on recording EMG activity in identifying REM sleep was established.

FUN FACT: In his book "The Promise of Sleep," William C Dement mentioned that when he proposed the idea of recording a woman's REM sleep, Professor Kleitman wholly opposed it. In fact, it was only after Dement's marriage that he was permitted to record the sleep of a woman: his own wife! [9].

Sleep Staging and Scoring: Then and Now

After the pioneer work of staging the sleep as non-REM and REM by William Dement, a committee specializing in sleep scoring headed by Allan Rechtschaffen and Anthony Kales, in 1967, conceptualized the very first universal sleep scoring system, commonly referred to as R&K or Rechtschaffen and Kales [10]. Using a central EEG, chin EMG, two channels of EOG, and an epoch-by-epoch approach (epochs of 20 or 30 s), they scored sleep in five different stages: stage 1, 2, 3, 4, and REM on paper. The guidelines under R&K system were designed for normal sleep patterns, and the limitation of the system became clear with increasing recognition of various sleep disorders [11]. Over the years, many changes have been made to this system, and it was in 2007, when the American Academy of Sleep Medicine (AASM) published The AASM Manual for the Scoring of Sleep and Associated Events. Not only did it revise the R&K sleep staging, but also addressed the digital platform for recording cardio-respiratory monitoring, sleep-related movement disorders, scoring of arousals, besides the basic EEG, EMG, and EOG, in all age groups [12]. Sleep is still scored in five different stages, but the terminologies describing them have been updated as: Stage W (wakefulness), N1 (NREM 1 sleep), N2 (NREM 2 sleep), N3 (NREM 3 sleep), and R (REM sleep) [13].

Polysomnography Today

In today's time and age, digital polygraphs with the capability of recording 16 channels or more of data have almost completely replaced the paper based analog four channel studies. The computerized data acquisition and storage allows the recording of various functions during a polysomnography, ideally including: EEG, EOG, mental/submental EMG, limb muscle activity (bilateral tibialis anterior EMG, to detect movement of the legs), EKG, respiratory effort, airflow, snoring, peripheral pulse oximetry, body positioning, and uninterrupted video recording. Special techniques, like measuring the intraesophageal pressure, esophageal pH; and penile tumescence for the assessment of erectile dysfunction during the polysomnography are not routinely used [5, 14].

Technical Considerations

The equipment for recording the polysomnographic activity utilizes a series of amplifiers (both alternating current–AC, direct current–DC) with varied (high and low) frequency filters and sensitivity settings. The differential amplifiers with appropriate filters amplify the difference between two electrodes, while simultaneously subtracting the undesirable potentials like galvanic skin response, DC electrode imbalance, and environmental noise reflected onto the EEG, EMG, or EOG channel, eventually recording a non-contaminated specific band of interest. This ability of the amplifiers to eliminate the extraneous signal is quantified by the common mode rejection ratio (CMRR), which in most of the PSG settings is set in excess of 10,000 to 1 [14].

The two main filters used in PSG are: a low-frequency filter (also known as a high-pass filter) attenuating lower frequencies, and a high-frequency filter (also known as a low-pass filter) which attenuates higher frequencies. The higher frequency physiological parameters like electroencephalogram (EEG), electrooculogram (EOG), electromyogram (EMG), and the electrocardiogram (ECG) are recorded using the differential AC amplifiers. On the other hand, DC amplifiers have no low-frequency filters and typically assist in recording CPAP titration pressure changes, intraesophageal pressure readings, esophageal pH output, and the output from the pulse oximeter. To record respiratory flow and effort, either AC or DC amplifiers can be used. In addition to the above filters, a 60-Hz notch filter is present in most of the PSG amplifiers. It helps attenuate the 60-Hz artifact, which otherwise, can easily contaminate an EEG recording. This filter, however, should be sparingly used, as it can attenuate some prime components of the recording, like muscle activity and epileptiform spikes [14].

Now that we have an idea of the filters used in a PSG study, let's address another important setting—Sensitivity. It is usually expressed in millivolts per centimeter or microvolts per millimeter. With the sensitivity switch, tiny voltages generated by the eyes, heart, and the cerebral cortex can be transformed into an interpretable form. These switches should be set to record a sufficient amplitude for interpretation. Current recommendations on sensitivity for each channel can be found on AASM's website.

Polysomnography: The Recording

In this section, we will look at the basic set up of a sleep laboratory, variables (EEG, EOG, and EMG), their calibrations, and the various montages involved during a PSG study.

Sleep Laboratory/Sleep Center

A sleep laboratory should have comfortable room, in a calmer area, free from noise and with an optimal room temperature. The room settings should be able to help the patient relax and fall asleep. Some patients might feel comfortable if they are allowed to bring in their home pillows, sleepwear, and a book to read. At the end of the day, for a successful sleep study, it is imperative for the patient to have a sound sleep on the day of the study.

Once the patient is comfortable, the electrodes should be hooked up. Electrodes are generally used to record EEG, EOG, EMG, ECG, and sometimes respiratory effort. The first step in placing the electrodes is identifying the sites for placement, using the International Ten-Twenty System [15]. They should be placed in such a way, that they record the maximum waveform amplitude possible, with minimal to zero impedance. Lower the impedance, higher would be the conductance, and the amplitude waveforms. To achieve lowest possible impedance, the sleep technologist should scrub the area where the electrodes will be placed. It is important to match the impedance of all electrodes to avoid artifacts [14].

The sleep lab should have the option of video recording to monitor the sleep behaviors. Using a low light/infrared camera, it is possible to obtain good quality video in the dark. The camera should be mounted across from the head end of the bed to give a good view.

Recording Variables

The standard speed for recording a standard PSG is 10 mm/s, but for easier identification of epileptiform activities, a speed of 30 mm/s is used. This section deals with the variables involved in a standard PSG recording.

Electroencephalography

Electroencephalography is the summation of excitatory postsynaptic potentials (EPSP) and inhibitory postsynaptic potentials (IPSP) recorded over the scalp electrodes. The ideal electrodes used in EEG are the silver-silver chloride electrodes and the gold cup electrodes. The only catch with silver-silver chloride electrodes is that they need repeated chloriding for maintenance.

The electrodes are applied onto the scalp with the help of electrode paste or conducting gel, in a pattern determined by the 10–20 system. According to the original R-K scoring system, only one channel (C3-A2 or C4-A1) was recommended. However, many of the laboratories use a minimum of four channels (C3-A2, C4-A1, O1-A1, O2-A2) to demonstrate the onset of sleep. These standard recommended EEG recordings of 1–4 channels of recordings may miss most of the epileptiform discharges. Therefore, it was concluded that a PSG study should include multiple channels of EEG covering temporal and parasagittal regions in patients suspected of having epilepsy in sleep.

The landmarks for placing the electrodes include the nasion, the inion, and the left and right preauricular points. All the electrodes are positioned with respect to these landmark points.

Once the electrodes are placed, then all the electrode wires from the scalp are secured into a ponytail at the back of the head, terminating in one common pin, and this is plugged into an electrode box, called a *JACK*. The wires from the *Jack box* are connected to an electrode montage selector through a shielded conductor cable [13, 16, 17].

Scalp electrodes → Jack box → Electrode montage selector.

Electroencephalography Patterns: The Normal, the Abnormal, and the Mimickers

The Normal Pattern

During wakefulness, the dominant rhythm in adults is an alpha rhythm (8–13 Hz), which is symmetric and synchronous over the parieto-occipital regions, commonly referred to as "posterior dominant rhythm" or "posterior alpha rhythm." This rhythm is best noticed in a quiet wakeful state with eyes closed and is attenuated significantly when the eyes are open. In a small number of normal adults, the dominant rhythm is a low-amplitude beta frequency (greater than 13 Hz), but in a majority of them, the beta rhythms can be appreciated mostly in the frontal and the central regions, intermixed with the posterior alpha rhythm. EEG rhythms vary according to the stages of sleep (wakefulness to NREM to REM). In older adults, a few normal variations do occur, like progressive slowing of the alpha rhythm, lower amplitude delta waves, sleep fragmentation with early morning awakenings, and multiple sleep stage shifts [13, 16].

The Abnormal Pattern

Certain abnormal patterns on the EEG tend to have a strong predilection towards epilepsy. These waveforms of spikes, sharp waves, spike and waves, sharp- and slow-wave complexes, and rhythmic focal activities in neonatal seizures suggest epileptiform patterns. A spike waveform appears suddenly out of the background rhythm, lasting for about 20–70 ms and often terminates with an after-going slow wave. A sharp waveform is similar to the spike waveform in all aspects, except the duration (70–200 ms). Classically, a true epileptiform spike or sharp wave is a biphasic or triphasic wave with a sharp ascent, immediately followed by a slow descent, and the amplitude is about 30% higher than the monophasic background rhythm. Spike and waves, sharp- and slow-wave complexes can be transient or repetitive. In patients with suspected seizure disorders, certain procedures are done to aid seizure activation like sleep deprivation, hyperventilation, and photic stimulation. Tonic-clonic seizures can have sudden bursts of spike and slow waves which are symmetrical and synchronous, start at 4–6 Hz, gradually slow down and eventually stop. Absence seizures are also symmetrical and synchronous, but are 3 Hz frontal spike and wave discharges. The interictal pattern may show generalized 4–6 Hz spike- and slow-wave discharges or multiple spike and waves [16].

The Mimickers

There are certain non-epileptiform patterns that may mimic epileptiform waveforms. These include sharp artifacts, sharp transients during sleep and wakefulness, and epileptiform-like patterns without epileptogenic significance.

Sharp Artifacts

These include electrocardiograph artifacts, muscle artifacts, and electrode pops. EKG artifacts can be identified by the morphology, rhythm, and synchrony with simultaneously recorded EKG.

Muscle artifacts can be resolved by getting the patient to relax.

Electrode pop artifacts are due to a faulty electrode contact and are resolved after the electrode issue is fixed.

Sharp Transients Seen During Sleep and Wakefulness

These include Mu rhythm, K-complexes, sharp appearing spindles, positive occipital sharp transients (POSTS), posterior slow waves of youth, vertex sharp waves, benign epileptiform transients of sleep (BETS) or small sharp spikes (SSS), hypnagogic or hypnopompic hypersynchrony, photic driving responses resembling spikes or sharp waves. These transients vary by distribution, morphology, patient's alertness, and the background.

Mu rhythm is a brief burst of 7–11 Hz over the central regions (C3–C4 electrodes) bilaterally, and attenuates on intention to move or actual movement of the limbs.

The K-complex is characterized by a high-voltage negative positive potential followed by sleep spindles. Sharp sleep spindles or sigma waves are sinusoidal waves with a frequency of 11–16 Hz and together with K-complexes form the hallmark of NREM sleep.

Positive occipital sharp transients (POSTS) of sleep are seen predominantly in stage I and II NREM. They are characterized by bilateral monophasic positive polarity in posterior temporal and occipital electrodes.

Posterior slow waves of youth are the 2–3 Hz slow waves superimposed on occipital alpha rhythm bilaterally, which attenuate on opening the eyes. They are common between ages 2 and 21 years.

Vertex sharp waves are basically negative potentials around the vertex and can spread to adjoining areas too.

Benign epileptiform transients of sleep (BETS) or small sharp spikes (SSS) are best recorded in the ipsilateral ear montage during stage I NREM.

Hypnogogic hypersynchrony is characterized by brief bursts of synchronous high-voltage slow (4–5 Hz) activity. It is a well-recognized normal variant of drowsiness, usually seen in children aged 3 months–13 years. Hypnagogic hypersynchrony and posterior slow wave of youth are age dependent.

Sometimes, several spikes like waves are located in the temporal regions, called wicket rhythms. These may be mistaken for epileptiform discharges [16, 18].

Epileptiform-Like Patterns Without Epileptogenic Significance

These include periodic or pseudoperiodic lateralized epileptiform discharges (PLEDs), triphasic waves, burst suppression, subclinical rhythmic epileptiform discharge of adults, and periodic complexes. Further discussion of these is beyond the scope of this chapter.

Electromyography

Electromyography (EMG) is an essential component of the polysomnogram. Not only does it aid in sleep staging, but also for the diagnosis and classification of sleep disorders. It denotes the summation of the electrical activity on many individual motor units in a muscle as a result of depolarization. Normally, there is a basic tone in the muscles during awake state and NREM sleep, but this tone is significantly diminished or absent in the majority of the muscles in REM sleep. The patterns seen in REM sleep may be tonic, rhythmic, or dystonic and phasic. Dystonic patterns last for 500–1000 ms or longer. Rhythmic patterns are recorded in patients with tremors. Phasic patterns can be myoclonic bursts, which last for a duration of 20–500 ms characteristically in REM sleep, or can be EMG patterns which are in phase with inspiratory bursts.

A gold cup or silver-silver chloride electrode is classically used to record EMGs from mentalis or submentalis and the right and left tibialis anterior muscles. The mental or submental EMG records the axial muscle tone and is essential for the diagnosis of REM sleep, as the axial muscle tone is diminished in it. While recording a chin EMG, a minimum of three electrodes are applied so that in case of any artifacts in one of the electrodes, the additional one can be utilized without compromising on the patient's sleep. Sometimes, an additional electrode is placed over the masseter muscle to record the EMG activity during bruxism (tooth grinding).

The tibialis electrodes aid in recording the periodic limb movements (PLMS) in sleep. The recording for PLMS should also include one or two electrodes in the upper limb muscles. In patients with suspected REM sleep behavior disorder (RBD), electrodes are placed on the extensor digitorum muscles in the upper limbs, in addition to the regular tibialis electrodes.

When the electrodes are placed on the limbs, the ideal distance of separation is 2–2.5 cm.

Intercostal EMG is usually recorded from the seventh to ninth intercostal spaces, along with electrodes for monitoring the diaphragmatic activity. An ideal EMG would show a progressive reduction of the tone from a wakeful state to NREM to an almost complete absence of tone in REM sleep. In certain disorders like REM sleep behavior disorder, this atonia in REM sleep is absent and is replaced by phasic burst patterns [13, 14].

Electrooculography

In the eye, the cornea is relatively positive compared to the retina, which is relatively negative, creating a dipole. So when an eye movement occurs, the orientation of this dipole changes and this movement is demonstrated on the electrooculography (EOG). It is actually a measure of the corneo-retinal potential difference and not the eye muscle potential changes. Just like in EEG and EMG, gold cup or silver-silver chloride electrodes are used to record the EOG. Ideally, electrodes are placed 1 cm on the outer canthus of the right eye (ROC) superiorly and laterally, and 1 cm on the outer canthus of the left eye (LOC) inferiorly and laterally. Both ROC and LOC are then connected to a reference electrode, on the mastoid process. ROC and LOC are now referred to as A1 and A2, respectively. In addition to these electrodes, infraorbital and supraorbital electrodes can be attached to reinforce the proper recording of vertical eye movements, which is imperative in the multiple sleep latency test (MSLT).

Waking eye movements (WEMs), slow eye movements (SEMs), and rapid eye movements (REMs) are recorded in an EOG. WEMs include blinking of the eyes, reading eye movements, and saccadic eye movements. SEMs are recorded in the horizontal axis during the NREM sleep and progressively disappear in the deeper stages of sleep. REMs appear in bursts in all directions (horizontal, vertical, and oblique) during the REM sleep, but more common in the horizontal axis [13, 19].

Electrocardiography

Two gold cup electrodes, one over the sternum and the other on the lateral chest, are sufficient to record the EKG during the polysomnography. These electrodes can pick up brady-, tachyarrhythmias, or any other arrhythmias commonly encountered in patients with obstructive sleep apnea syndrome (OSAS) [14].

Respiration: The Effort and the Airflow

Respiratory monitoring of the airflow and effort during PSG is essential for the diagnosis of apneas, hypopneas, respiratory effort related arousals (RERAs), and other sleep-related breathing disorders. In clinical practice, piezoelectric strain gauges and respiratory inductive plethysmography aid in monitoring the respiratory effort.

Strain gauges are belts placed around the chest and abdomen to detect the movements with respiration. The disadvantage of strain gauges is their inability to differentiate central from obstructive sleep apneas, and also being displaced by body movements, eventually leading to an inaccurate measurement.

Respiratory inductive plethysmography (RIP) utilizes transducers to measure changes in the thoraco-abdominal cross-sectional areas during breathing. The summation of these two compartments is proportional to the airflow. Just like strain gauges, these transducers can be displaced by body movements, causing inaccurate measurements. The gold standard to measure respiratory effort is by intraesophageal pressure monitoring. Diagnosis of upper airway resistance, classification of apneas and hypopneas are some of the indications for intraesophageal pressure monitoring.

Other techniques like impedance pneumography, respiratory magnetometers, and the previously described intercostal and diaphragmatic EMGs have been used unsuccessfully.

Thermistors, thermocouples, and nasal cannula-pressure transducers have been used to record the airflow. Both thermistors and thermocouples deal with temperature variations in the airflow, and neither of them are as sensitive as nasal pressure transducers in detecting airflow limitations and hypopneas. Nasal pressure monitoring uses the principle of alternate decrement and increment of nasal pressure during inspiration and expiration, respectively, indirectly estimating the airflow. One of the major limitations of nasal pressure monitoring is that it cannot measure airflow in mouth breathers and is rendered ineffective in nasal obstruction.

Capnography estimates the intra-alveolar carbon dioxide (CO_2), through the quantification of the expired CO_2 in the airflow and also the partial pressure of CO_2 in the alveoli. It is considered as the best noninvasive method to detect alveolar hypoventilation. The drawback of this study is the high costs involved, but it is still used in children with a suspicion of obstructive sleep apnea.

To detect the arterial oxygen content (PaO_2), the best way is by an invasive arterial cannula, which is not viable practically. Therefore, finger pulse oximetry is the standard to monitor arterial oxygen saturation (SaO_2) or oxyhemoglobin saturation. This information provides an estimate of the level of respiratory dysfunction [14, 20].

Body Positioning and Snoring

In patients with suspected OSA, it is important to monitor the body position while titrating for the optimal continuous positive airway pressure (CPAP), as snoring and apneas are common in supine posture.

To quantitatively record snoring, a tiny microphone can be placed on the patient's neck.

Gastroesophageal Studies

When patients present with issues related to gastroesophageal reflux, then a specialized procedure monitoring the esophageal pH with a pH probe can be performed to demonstrate the reflux and its correlation with EEG arousals or other physiological events. Patients can have severe chest pain due to gastroesophageal reflux and cause an arousal from sleep, which can be mistaken for sleep apnea. Usually the pH probe is swallowed, and the pH is monitored at the level of the distal esophagus [14].

Indications for Polysomnography

Approved clinical indications for an overnight PSG study suggested by the AASM include sleep-disordered breathing, positive airway pressure titration in sleep-disordered breathing, overnight PSG with MSLT for narcolepsy, atypical or unusual parasomnias, sleep-related seizure-disorder assessment, evaluation of OSAS before undergoing laser-assisted uvulopalatopharyngoplasty (LAUP), and a follow-up PSG to assess the treatment benefits [18]. Routine polysomnography is not recommended for simple parasomnias.

Peripheral Arterial Tonometry

Using a finger bound plethysmograph, peripheral arterial tonometry (PAT) measures the peripheral arterial tone. The peripheral arterial tone is dictated by peripheral blood pressure, sympathetic activity, and by the peripheral resistance of the vessels. In patients with obstructive sleep apnea, the apneic episodes are associated with an arousal from sleep. These respiration-triggered arousals increase the sympathetic activity, which indirectly raises the peripheral arterial tone. This increased tone is measured via the pulse-related arterial filling at the tip of the finger [21, 22]. WatchPAT system (Itamar Medical, Ltd., Israel) uses the above principle in conjunction with other body parameters (pulse oximetry, heart rate, and actigraphy) in an algorithm to determine apnea/hypopnea index (AHI) and respiratory disturbance index (RDI) [23].

This was first conceptualized as an inexpensive alternative to the conventional sleep study with a polysomnogram. The mean cost of a PAT and PSG was US$ 895.74 and US$ 2252.73, respectively [21]. In a recent meta-analysis, it was demonstrated that the distribution of sleep states and respiratory indexes calculated using peripheral arterial tonometry had a higher degree of correlation with that of a classic polysomnogram [22]. Also, the simplistic procedure of a PAT with the patient having to wear reduced number of leads automatically increases patient comfort levels. In view of these events, PAT devices should be considered as a viable alternative to PSG for the diagnosis of OSAS.

1 The Basics of Polysomnography

Calibrations

Physiologic calibration along with the calibration of the PSG equipment needs to be performed prior to the initiation of the sleep testing. The first step in equipment calibration is to run an all-channel calibration followed by individual channel calibration.

For the physiologic calibration, certain procedures are performed after connecting the electrodes and other monitors. The procedures include opening and closing eyes, clenching the jaw, inhaling and exhaling, and flexing the hands and feet. Backup electrodes should also be tested during this calibration [14, 20].

Montages

The pattern of arrangement of different channels is called a montage. While some sleep studies require a limited number of channels, others require extra channels. Tables 1.1, 1.2, 1.3, 1.4, 1.5, and 1.6 outline the typical montages used in different sleep studies.

Table 1.1 Montage for standard polysomnogram [14]

Channel	Name
1	F3-A2
2	F4-A1
3	C3-A2
4	C4-A1
5	O1-A2
6	O2-A1
7	LEOG
8	REOG
9	Chin-EMG
10	LAT-EMG
11	RAT-EMG
12	Nasal/oral airflow
13	Nasal pressure
14	Snore1-Snore2
15	Thoracic motion
16	Abdominal motion
17	Backup motion
18	Intercostal EMG
19	EKG
20	SaO_2

LEOG and REOG left and right electrooculogram, *LAT and RAT-EMG* left and right anterior tibialis surface EMG, *EKG* electrocardiogram, *Snore1-Snore2* monitor the snoring, *thoracic and abdominal motion* records respiratory effort, *Nasal/oral airflow* record the airflow, SaO_2 arterial oxygen saturation via pulse oximetry, *Pes* intrathoracic (esophageal) pressure monitor

Table 1.2 Montage for CPAP trial

Channel	Name
1	F3-A2
2	F4-A1
3	C3-A2
4	C4-A1
5	O1-A2
6	O2-A1
7	LEOG
8	REOG
9	Chin-EMG
10	LAT-EMG
11	RAT-EMG
12	Oral airflow
13	Mask flow
14	Tidal volume
15	Snore1-Snore2
16	Thoracic motion
17	Abdominal motion
18	Backup motion
19	EKG
20	SaO_2

Table 1.3 Montage for intrathoracic pressure monitoring

Channel	Name
1	F3-A2
2	F4-A1
3	C3-A2
4	C4-A1
5	O1-A2
6	O2-A1
7	LEOG
8	REOG
9	Chin-EMG
10	LAT-EMG
11	RAT-EMG
12	Nasal/oral airflow
13	Nasal pressure
14	Snore1-Snore2
15	Thoracic motion
16	Abdominal motion
17	Backup motion
18	Intercostal EMG
19	EKG
20	SaO_2
21	Pes

1 The Basics of Polysomnography

Table 1.4 Montage for seizures or suspected parasomnias

Channel	Name
1	Fp1-F7
2	F7-T3
3	T3-T5
4	T5-O1
5	Fp1-F3
6	F3-C3
7	C3-P3
8	P3-O1
9	Fp2-F4
10	F4-C4
11	C4-P4
12	P4-O2
13	Fp2-F8
14	F8-T4
15	T4-T6
16	T6-O2
17	F3-A2
18	F4-A1
19	C3-A2
20	C4-A1
21	O1-A2
22	O2-A1
23	LEOG
24	REOG
25	Chin-EMG
26	LAT-EMG
27	RAT-EMG
28	Nasal/oral airflow
29	Nasal pressure
30	Snore1-Snore2
31	Thoracic motion
32	Abdominal motion
33	Backup motion
34	Intercostal EMG
35	EKG
36	SaO_2

Table 1.5 Montage for REM sleep behavior disorder

Channel	Name
1	Fp1-F7
2	F7-T3
3	T3-T5
4	T5-O1
5	Fp1-F3
6	F3-C3
7	C3-P3
8	P3-O1
9	Fp2-F4
10	F4-C4
11	C4-P4
12	P4-O2
13	Fp2-F8
14	F8-T4
15	T4-T6
16	T6-O2
17	F3-A2
18	F4-A1
19	C3-A2
20	C4-A1
21	O1-A2
22	O2-A1
23	LEOG
24	REOG
25	Chin-EMG
26	LAT-EMG
27	RAT-EMG
28	LAT1-EMG
29	RAT1-EMG
30	LED-EMG
31	RED-EMG
32	Nasal/oral airflow
33	Nasal pressure
34	Snore1-Snore2
35	Thoracic motion
36	Abdominal motion
37	Backup motion
38	Intercostal EMG
39	EKG
40	SaO_2

Table 1.6 Montage for multiple sleep latency test

Channel	Name
1	F3-A2
2	F4-A1
3	C3-A2
4	C4-A1
5	O1-A2
6	O2-A1
7	LEOG
8	REOG
9	Chin-EMG
10	LAT-EMG
11	RAT-EMG
12	EKG

Types of Sleep Studies

There are numerous types of sleep studies that can be performed based on the sleep disorder in question.

(a) *Nocturnal Polysomnogram (NPSG):* It is the gold standard amongst the various sleep studies used to diagnose sleep disorders, like sleep apnea, sleep-related hypoxia/hypoventilation, periodic limb movement disorders, etc. Multiple physiological variables such as EEG, EMG, EOG, EKG, respiratory effort and airflow, oxygen saturation, and snoring [22]. These variables and the sleep montage used for PSG have already been discussed earlier in this chapter.

(b) *Continuous Positive Airway Pressure (CPAP) Titration:* After the diagnosis of obstructive sleep apnea syndrome (OSAS) has been established by polysomnography, the patient undergoes CPAP titration to determine the most effective pressure in decimating the apneic events and snoring. The sleep montage for CPAP titration has been described earlier in this chapter.

(c) *Split Study:* In patients with severe sleep apnea, a split study combining a 2–4 h diagnostic test and a therapeutic test on the same night can be performed to avoid a delay in initiating the treatment. Sometimes, the patient may return for the therapeutic CPAP titration on the consecutive night of nocturnal PSG.

(d) *Bi-Level Titration:* Some patients with very severe OSAS or patients who are intolerant of CPAP, pressures on inhalation, and an alternate pressure on exhalation are titrated to ease the breathing.

(e) *NPSG with End-Tidal CO_2:* End-tidal CO_2 monitoring during a NPSG aids in the detection of hypercapnia and obesity hypoventilation. This is the gold standard in pediatric polysomnography.

(f) *REM Behavior Disorder (RBD):* Electrodes are attached to both arms and legs to record the movements during REM sleep. This can help diagnose if a patient is acting out the dreams at night.
(g) *Multiple Sleep Latency Test (MSLT):* This is a study used to identify the presence of narcolepsy after a full night's sleep, usually performed during the day after a nocturnal PSG. MSLT has a wide application in basic, clinical, and pharmacological sleep research. This test has been standardized by the AASM and includes both general and specific procedures. Keeping a log of the patient's sleep, along with avoidance of stimulants and REM suppressing medications for at least 2 weeks are some of the general procedures done before the test. Before beginning the test, physiologic calibrations are performed, and then the patient is asked to fall asleep. The actual test is a series of five nap opportunities, 2 h apart, and each session lasts for a maximum of 20 min, and the patients should remain awake between sessions. Variables used in this study include EEG, EOG, submentalis EMG, tibialis anterior EMG, and EKG. Sleep-onset rapid eye movements (SOREMs) and mean sleep latency are measured in this study. SOREM is defined as the occurrence of REM sleep within 15 min of sleep onset. Mean sleep latency is averaged from the sum of latency to sleep onset from each of the five nap sessions. Normal mean sleep latency is about 10–15 min. Excessive sleepiness is defined by a mean sleep onset latency of 8 min or less [14, 24, 25, 26].
(h) MSLT is most commonly indicated in the diagnosis of narcolepsy, which is characterized by a mean sleep latency of <8 min, along with SOREMs in two or more of the five nap sessions during the MSLT. If there is a SOREM period in the preceding baseline sleep study, this can be counted towards the required two SOREMs for the diagnosis of Narcolepsy. MSLT is not routinely indicated in OSAS. But in patients with OSAS who continue to have excessive daytime sleepiness (EDS) despite optimal therapy, it is important to think of narcolepsy as a differential, as both narcolepsy and OSAS can co-exist. MSLT's diagnostic yield increases with repeat testing [27].
(i) *Maintenance of Wakefulness Test (MWT):* This is slightly different from MSLT and measures an individual's ability to resist sleep and stay awake. It is commonly used for assessing "fitness for duty" in patients post sleep-related accidents or a sleep disorder with excessive sleepiness constituting a hazard to personal or public safety. AASM recommends a total of four trials at 2-h intervals, with the duration of each trial lasting for 40 min. Ideally, the test is performed 1–3 h after the patient's wake-up time and does not require an overnight PSG. Calibrations and the montage are similar to the ones used in MSLT. Sleep onset and mean sleep latency are measured by MWT. Sleep onset is the time from the start of the recording to the onset of three consecutive stage I NREM epochs, or one epoch of any other sleep stage. Mean sleep latency <8 min is deemed abnormal. The other indication besides assessment of "fitness for duty," is testing the efficacy of the treatment of a sleep disorder (stimulants in narcolepsy, CPAP in OSAS) [14, 24, 26, 28].
(j) *Actigraphy:* Using the principle of reduced movements during sleep and increased movements during wakefulness, actigraphy aids in the evaluation of

many circadian rhythm disorders like delayed sleep phase syndrome, advanced sleep phase syndrome, non-24-h sleep-wake syndrome, blindness-related dyssomnia, and jet lag. Circadian rhythm disorders show misalignments between active-inactive periods, desired bed time, and clock time. It can also estimate total sleep time, when PSG is not available.
(k) An actigraph contains an internal clock, a digital memory device, event markers, accelerometers, often includes a photo sensor, and resembles a digital watch. It has to be worn continuously for about a week or more, on the nondominant wrist, while simultaneously maintaining a sleep diary. Once the patient returns the actigraph, the data can be extracted onto the computer and analyzed [14, 24, 26].
(l) *Home sleep testing (HST):* This was approved in 2008 by Center for Medicare Services as an acceptable diagnostic procedure for sleep apnea. It does not help in diagnosing sleep disorders other than sleep apnea. HST records cardiopulmonary data using a Holter-type device, intended for unattended use at home. The recorders are classified as levels II, III, and IV, with type III (cardiopulmonary) being the most common type. Most of the recorded measures are derived from the ones used in a standard PSG (temperature transducers or nasal pressure sensors, finger oximetry, diaphragm movement), but some unique measurements (peripheral arterial tonometry, forehead reflectance oximetry and EEG, accelerometers on the legs, and transformed breathing sounds) are used by certain HST devices.
(m) Any patient with five or more apnea or hypopnea ($\geq 4\%$ oxyhemoglobin desaturation) index (AHI) on HST qualifies for positive airway pressure. In patients with co-morbid conditions like hypertension, heart disease, impaired cognition, history of stroke, positive pressure can be given for AHI ≥ 5. The drawbacks of HST are pretty obvious; since it is an unattended study, it is more prone to patient tampering and data loss, along with the patient needing assistance in case of troubleshooting. Therefore, HST can rule in sleep apnea, but not rule out. Patients who do not meet the diagnostic criteria for OSA can be given the option of a repeat HST or they can be scheduled for a polysomnography in the sleep laboratory. Another important limitation of the HST is its inability to identify "Respiratory effort related arousals" (RERAs) [26, 29].

Pediatric Polysomnogram

The physiological variables during pediatric polysomnography are identical to the ones measured during polysomnography in adults, with a few noted exceptions. The AASM recommends the following:

(a) EEG: F4-M1, C4-M1, and O2-M1 and F3-M2, C3-M2, and O1-M2 on the contralateral side.
(b) EMG: submental and bilateral tibial
(c) EOG: right and left
(d) Nasal pressure

(e) Oronasal airflow (thermistry)
(f) EKG
(g) SaO_2 with pulse waveform
(h) Thorax and abdominal wall motion
(i) End-tidal PCO_2
(j) Body position monitor
(k) Snoring microphone (optional)
(l) Video

EEG monitoring will need a sensitivity of 10–15 μV/mm instead of the regular adult 7 μV/mm, as children have high amplitude brainwaves. For the airflow and the effort, in addition to the standard equipment, a sensor for oral breathing is needed as many children breathe through their mouth due to enlarged adenoids. In the pediatric population, end-tidal CO_2 is overly sensitive as a measure for airflow. Therefore, it is used only as an indicator of hypoventilation and not obstruction. End-tidal CO_2 is measured from a nasal cannula, or from an endotracheal or tracheostomy tube. An alternative to end-tidal CO_2 as a measure for hypoventilation is transcutaneous PCO_2, which is especially beneficial in children on CPAP, as CPAP interferes with end-tidal CO_2 measurement. In children, body position plays a minimal role in OSAS. Finally, the most important part of the polysomnography is having a video monitor to assist in the diagnoses of parasomnias, seizures, apneic events, etc. [30].

How Is It Different from Adult Sleep Scoring?

Anders et al. described a set of criteria for infants younger than 2 months of age, which are invariably used [31]. In infants, the sleep has three states: active sleep, quiet sleep, and indeterminate sleep. Infants usually enter sleep with active sleep (equivalent to REM sleep in adults), and this makes up for about 50% of the total sleep time. Active sleep can show phasic bursts of facial motor activity (smiles, sucking, frowning), body movements, vocalization, in addition to increased heart rate variability, irregular respiration, and diminished EMG activity. Quiet sleep is characterized by a lower heart rate, deeper unlabored breathing, increased EMG activity, behavioral silence, and lack of movements. Indeterminate sleep is all the epochs that do not correlate with active or quiet sleep. By the age of 6 months, sleep in infants can be scored by the adult NREM (N1, N2, and N3).

With increasing age, the EEG patterns also change. The pediatric EEG is usually a higher amplitude, with a slower posterior dominant rhythm. Sleep spindles are first observed at 2–3 months; K-complexes at 4–6 months; slow-wave activity at 4–5 months, and then become prominent thereafter. The amount of slow-wave sleep and REM change drastically from infancy into adolescence [30].

Respiratory scoring for children up to 17 years is different from adults. Kids usually have a higher respiratory rate, lower functional residual capacity, and as a result of this end up desaturating from brief apneas. That is the reason we score apneas and hypopneas if they are at least two breaths duration, even if the duration is ≤10 s (the standard duration in adults). Central apneas are more common in REM sleep and are scored only if they are longer than 20 s, or shorter and associated with ≥3% desaturation or arousal. Hypopneas in pediatrics are a 50% reduction in airflow with either ≥3% desaturation or arousal. In children, an apnea hypopnea index (AHI) index in the range of 2–5/h calls for treatment [30].

Sometimes, instead of the classical apneas and hypopneas, obstructive hypoventilation with hypercapnia, snoring, and paradoxical breathing occurs in children. Since the majority of obstructive events occur in REM sleep, it is imperative to obtain a polysomnogram with sufficient REM sleep.

Adults have a lower threshold for arousals, compared to children. That is why children can have obstructive episodes without an arousal on EEG.

Key Points

1. Polysomnogram a.k.a sleep study is a comprehensive study of the patient's sleep that acquires information from various channels including scalp EEG, chest and abdominal movements, EKG, EMG from limbs, and pulse/oximeter.
2. During wakefulness, the dominant rhythm in adults is an alpha rhythm (8–13 Hz), which is symmetric and synchronous over the parieto-occipital regions, commonly referred to as "posterior dominant rhythm" or "posterior alpha rhythm." This rhythm is best noticed in a quiet wakeful state with eyes closed and is attenuated significantly when the eyes are open.
3. Approved clinical indications for an overnight PSG study suggested by the AASM include sleep-disordered breathing, positive airway pressure titration in sleep-disordered breathing, overnight PSG with MSLT for narcolepsy, atypical or unusual parasomnias, sleep-related seizure-disorder assessment, evaluation of OSAS before undergoing laser-assisted uvulopalatopharyngoplasty (LAUP), and a follow-up PSG to assess the treatment benefits.
4. Using a finger bound plethysmograph, peripheral arterial tonometry (PAT) measures the peripheral arterial tone. The peripheral arterial tone is dictated by peripheral blood pressure, sympathetic activity, and by the peripheral resistance of the vessels. Respiration-triggered arousals increase the sympathetic activity, which indirectly raises the peripheral arterial tone.
5. Physiologic calibration along with the calibration of the PSG equipment needs to be performed prior to the initiation of the sleep testing.
6. Multiple sleep latency test (MSLT) is done if there is a suspicion of narcolepsy. Presence of two episodes of sleep onset REM (SOREM) along with a shortened sleep onset latency is diagnostic of narcolepsy.
7. There are various different types of polysomnograms—diagnostic studies, PAP titration studies, split night studies, oxygen titration studies, etc. Home sleep studies are performed in patients who have a high probability of having sleep apnea. They lack the capacity to record EEG activity.
8. Maintainance of wakefulness test is done to measure one's capacity to stay awake.

References

1. Atkinson JW, editor. The evolution of polysomnographic technology. Philadelphia: Lippincott, Williams & Wilkins; 2007.
2. Caton R. The electric currents of the brain. Br Med J. 1875;2:278.
3. Deak M, Epstein LJ. The history of polysomnography. Sleep Med Clin. 2009;4(3):313–21.
4. Berger J. Uber das Elektrenkephalogramm des Menchen. Arch Psychiatr Nervenkr. 1929;87:527–70.
5. Haba-Rubio J, Krieger J. Evaluation instruments for sleep disorders: a brief history of polysomnography and sleep medicine. Introduction to modern sleep technology. Springer Nature. 2012. https://doi.org/10.1007/978-94-007-5470-6_2.
6. Aserinsky E, Kleitman N. Regularly occurring periods of eye motility, and concomitant phenomena, during sleep. Science. 1953;118(3062):273–4.
7. Jouvet M, Michel F, Courjon J. On a stage of rapid cerebral electrical activity in the course of physiological sleep. C R Seances Soc Biol Fil. 1959;153:1024–8.
8. Jouvet M, Mounier D. Effect of lesions of the pontile reticular formation on sleep in the cat. C R Seances Soc Biol Fil. 1960;154:2301–5.
9. Dement WC, editor. The promise of sleep. New York: Dell Publishing; 1999.
10. Rechtschaffen A, Kales A, editors. A manual of standardized terminology, techniques, and scoring system for sleep stages of human subjects. Washington, DC: Public Health Service, U.S. Government Printing Service; 1968.
11. Himanen SL, Hasan J. Limitations of Rechtschaffen and Kales. Sleep Med Rev. 2000;4(2):149–67.
12. Iber C, Ancoli-Israel S, Chesson A, Quan SF, for the American Academy of Sleep Medicine, editors. The AASM manual for the scoring of sleep and associated events: rules, terminology and technical specifications. Westchester: American Academy of Sleep Medicine; 2007.
13. Silber MH, Ancoli-Israel S, Bonnet MH, et al. The visual scoring of sleep in adults. J Clin Sleep Med. 2007;3(2):121–31.
14. Chokroverty S, Bhatt M, Goldhammer T. 1 - Polysomnographic recording technique. In: Atlas of sleep medicine. Philadelphia: Butterworth-Heinemann; 2005. p. 1–28. ISBN 9780750673983. https://doi.org/10.1016/B978-0-7506-7398-3.50005-X.
15. Jasper HH. The ten twenty electrode system of the International Federation. Electroenceph Clin Neurophysiol. 1958;10:371–5.
16. Chokroverty S, Bhatt M, Goldhammer T. 2 - Electroencephalography for the sleep specialists. In: Atlas of sleep medicine. Philadelphia: Butterworth-Heinemann; 2005. p. 29–93. ISBN 9780750673983. https://doi.org/10.1016/B978-0-7506-7398-3.50006-1.
17. Walczak T, Chokroverty S. Electroencephalography, electroymyography, and electrooculography: general principles and basic technology. In: Chokroverty S, editor. Sleep disorders medicine: basic science, technical considerations, and clinical aspects. 2nd ed. Boston: Butterworth Heinemann; 1999. p. 175–203.
18. Geyer J, Talathi S, Carney P. Introduction to sleep and polysomnography. In: Carney PR, Berry RB, Geyer JD, editors. Clinical sleep disorders. Philadelphia: Lippincott Williams & Wilkins; 2009. p. 265–6.
19. Chokroverty S. Role of electroencephalography in epilepsy. In: Chokroverty S, editor. Management of epilepsy. Boston: Butterworth-Heinemann; 1996. p. 67–112.
20. Keenan SA. Chapter 3 An overview of polysomnography. In: Guilleminault C, editor. Handbook of clinical neurophysiology, Vol. 6. Elsevier; 2005. p. 33–50. ISSN 1567-4231, ISBN 9780444515179. https://doi.org/10.1016/S1567-4231(09)70028-0.
21. Pinto JA, de Godoy LBM, Ribeiro RC, Mizoguchi EI, Hirsch LAM, Gomes LM. Accuracy of peripheral arterial tonometry in the diagnosis of obstructive sleep apnea. Braz J Otorhinolaryngol. 2015. https://doi.org/10.1016/j.bjorl.2015.07.005.

22. Yalamanchali S, Farajian V, Hamilton C, Pott TR, Samuelson CG, Friedman M. Diagnosis of obstructive sleep apnea by peripheral arterial tonometry. JAMA Otolaryngol Head Neck Surg. 2013. https://doi.org/10.1001/jamaoto.2013.5338.
23. Stuck BA, Maurer JT. Recent developments in the diagnosis and treatment of obstructive sleep apnea. HNO. 2016. https://doi.org/10.1007/s00106-016-0176-0.
24. Specialized Techniques. Atlas of sleep medicine. Elsevier BV; 2005. https://doi.org/10.1016/b978-0-7506-7398-3.50015-2
25. Afifi L, Kushida CA. Chapter 4 Multiple sleep latency test. In: Guilleminault C, editor. Handbook of clinical neurophysiology, Vol. 6. Elsevier; 2005. p. 51–57. ISSN 1567-4231, ISBN 9780444515179. https://doi.org/10.1016/S1567-4231(09)70029-2.
26. Hirshkowitz M. Chapter 3 - Introduction to sleep medicine diagnostics in adults. In: Barkoukis TJ, Matheson JK, Ferber R, Doghramji K, editors. Therapy in sleep medicine. Philadelphia: W. B. Saunders; 2012. p. 28–40. ISBN 9781437717037. https://doi.org/10.1016/B978-1-4377-1703-7.10003-9.
27. Practice parameters for clinical use of the multiple sleep latency tests and the maintenance of wakefulness test. An American Academy of Sleep Medicine report. Standards of Practice Committee of the American Academy of Sleep Medicine. Sleep 2005;28:113–121.
28. Doghramji K, Mitler MM. Chapter 5 The maintenance of wakefulness test. In: Guilleminault C, editor. Handbook of clinical neurophysiology, Vol. 6. Elsevier; 2005. p. 59–65. ISSN 1567-4231. ISBN 9780444515179. https://doi.org/10.1016/S1567-4231(09)70030-9.
29. Littner M, Hirshkowitz M, Sharafkhaneh A, Goodnight-White S. Nonlaboratory assessment of sleep-related breathing disorders. Sleep Med Clin. 2006;1:461–3.
30. Hoban TF. 13 - Pediatric polysomnography. In Chokroverty S, Bhatt M, Thomas RJ, editors. Atlas of sleep medicine. Philadelphia: Butterworth-Heinemann; 2005. p. 325–53. ISBN 9780750673983. https://doi.org/10.1016/B978-0-7506-7398-3.50017-6.
31. Anders T, Emdee A, et al. A manual of standardized terminology, techniques, and criteria for scoring of states of sleep and wakefulness in newborn infants. Los Angeles: UCLA Brain Information Service, NINDS Neurological Information Network; 1971.

Neuromuscular Respiratory Failure

Miguel Chuquilin and Nakul Katyal

The respiratory system consists of gas exchanging organs (the lungs) and a pump (chest wall, respiratory muscles, and central nervous system respiratory centers) that ventilates them. The act of breathing is very important for our survival and as such it is carefully regulated and coordinated. Respiratory failure can occur as a consequence of primary lung, breathing muscle, or central nervous system problems. Neuromuscular respiratory failure is the one that originates from weakness in the respiratory muscles.

In this chapter, we will discuss about basic concepts of anatomy and physiology of breathing, mechanisms of respiratory failure, clinical characteristics, evaluation, and predictors of the need for mechanical ventilation with focus on two of the most important ones, Guillain-Barré syndrome and myasthenia gravis.

Breathing Concepts

Anatomy and Physiology of the Respiratory Muscles

The respiratory system consists of the lungs and the respiratory muscles. The respiratory muscles can be divided into inspiratory and expiratory [1].

Inspiratory Muscles

These muscles include the diaphragm (the main muscle of inspiration), external intercostals, parasternal intercostals, and scalene muscles.

M. Chuquilin, M.D. (✉)
Department of Neurology, University of Florida, Gainesville, FL, USA
e-mail: miguel.chuquilin@neurology.ufl.edu

N. Katyal, M.D.
Department of Neurology, University of Missouri, Columbia, MO, USA

The diaphragm is responsible for 60–70% of the tidal volume in normal breathing [2]. It is dome-shaped and separates the thoracic and abdominal cavities. Its muscle fibers radiate from a central tendon and can be divided into two portions: crural diaphragm that inserts in the upper three lumbar vertebral bodies on the right and upper two lumbar bodies on the left, and costal diaphragm that inserts on the xiphoid process and on the inner surfaces of the lower six ribs and costal cartilages. The costal and crural fibers of the diaphragm contract independently of each other. When the diaphragm contracts, the thoracic cavity expands in a craniocaudal fashion. The costal diaphragmatic fibers also apply a force on the lower six ribs that lifts and rotates them outward [1, 3].

The diaphragm is innervated by the phrenic nerve (C3–5 fibers). Importantly, during normal (at rest) breathing, only type I (slow-twitch) and IIa (fast-twitch fatigue-resistant) diaphragmatic muscle fibers are preferentially recruited. Studies in rats and cats have shown that the force generated by the diaphragm (which can be approximated by measuring the transdiaphragmatic pressure (Pdi)) was only 20–30% of the maximum possible force obtained by bilateral phrenic nerve stimulation. In humans, eupneic Pdi is estimated to be 10% of maximum [4, 5]. On the other hand, during coughing or sneezing the force generation is near maximal and requires recruitment of all motor unit types (slow and fast-twitch), including type IIx and IIb fibers that are fatigue intermediate and fatigue-fast fibers but whose innervation ratio is larger and can generate greater force than type I and IIa fibers [5–7]. This makes sense as greater force is needed for coughing and sneezing.

The external intercostal muscles run downward in an oblique direction from each rib to the rib below. Because the lower insertion point of these muscles is more distant from the rib axis of rotation than the upper one, its contraction exerts greater torque on the lower rib, raising it with respect to the upper one and raising the rib cage [1, 8] (inspiratory effect).

The scalene muscles insert proximally in the anterior tubercles of the transverse processes of the lower five vertebrae and distally in the upper surface of the first rib (anterior and medius scalenes) and second rib (posterior scalene). They are innervated by C2–7 motoneurons. They used to be considered accessory muscles of inspiration, however, further studies have determined that these muscles are active even during inspiration at rest [3, 9] and for this reason they are considered inspiratory and not just accessory muscles.

The internal intercartilaginous intercostals (also called parasternal intercostals) are also active during quiet breathing in inspiration and are considered inspiratory muscles [8–10].

The sternocleidomastoid muscle inserts proximally in the mastoid process and occipital bone and distally in the manubrium sterni and medial part of the clavicle. It is innervated by the spinal accessory nerve (XI nerve). It is an accessory muscle of inspiration, active at high lung volumes or when there is a high ventilator demand such as during exercise [1, 3]. Other accessory inspiratory muscles include pectoralis, latissimus dorsi, erector spinae, and trapezius.

Expiratory Muscles

These muscles include the internal intercostals, and the four abdominal muscles (rectus abdominis, external oblique, internal oblique and transverse abdominis) [1].

At rest, expiration is mostly passive by recoil of the thoracic cage. Forceful expiration (e.g., for coughing) requires activation of the expiratory muscles [11].

The internal intercostals run downward and posteriorly in an oblique direction from one rib to the rib below. Because its lower insertion site is less distant from the ribs axis of rotation than the upper one, during their contraction they lower the ribs (expiratory effect) [1, 8, 9, 12].

Contraction of the abdominal muscles moves the abdominal wall inward, increasing intra-abdominal pressure which in turn moves the diaphragm upwards into the thoracic cavity (action mainly done by the internal and external obliques and transverse abdominis). Their contraction also pulls the lower ribs caudally (rectus, internal, and external obliques) and medially (external oblique and transverse), which deflates the ribcage. The abdominal muscles are the most important and powerful muscles of expiration [1, 3, 13].

Control of Breathing

Although breathing is done mostly automatically, we can also alter it voluntarily, for example, when taking a big breath, sniffing or when we hold our breath for a few seconds. There is evidence of direct corticospinal projections from the motor cortex to phrenic motoneurons that bypass the medulla [14]. Because the output of the inspiratory motoneurons depends on the result of descending and reflex inputs from different sources and can be altered by voluntary activity, these signals need to be integrated, possibly at the medulla or at the spinal cord [14].

Phrenic motor neurons are located in the ventral horn of cervical spinal segments C3–C5. These motor neuron discharges are driven primarily by bulbospinal inputs. Inspiratory phrenic motor neuron burst is driven by neurons located in the medullary rostral ventral respiratory group (rVRG) and dorsal respiratory group (DRG) [15]. The pre-Botzinger complex located caudal to the rVRG in the medulla has been identified as the central respiratory rhythm generator because it has pacemaker properties due to persistent Na^+ or Ca^{2+} currents [16]. The retrotrapezoid nucleus/parafacial respiratory group (RTN/pFRG) may serve as active expiratory rhythm generator (not for resting expiration) [17]. In addition to excitatory inputs associated with inspiration, phrenic motoneurons also receive inhibitory signals during the expiratory phase derived from the Botzinger complex in the rostral medulla [18, 19]. There are also cervical interneurons such as Renshaw cells or pre-phrenic cervical interneurons that can potentially modulate phrenic motoneuron response [15].

During breathing, there is a non-uniform activation of different motoneuron pools, which is required to achieve efficient ventilation. The drive is directed preferentially to those muscles or portions of muscles with the greatest mechanical advantage for inspiration [20]. The diaphragm and upper (third) dorsal external intercostal muscles are active earliest, before the onset of inspiratory flow and also have a higher average motor unit discharge rate than other main inspiratory muscles. The fifth dorsal external intercostal is recruited the latest in inspiration and its motor units discharge at lower firing rates. These different activation patterns in the intercostal muscles follow a principle called neuromechanical matching with differences in the timing and intensity of each motoneuron pool that correlate with each muscle ability to exert an inspiratory action (mechanical advantage), perhaps for metabolic reasons [8]. These differences in activation and firing rate are due to differences in inspiratory drive to each motor neuron pool. The motor units fire at higher frequencies in the rostral intercostal spaces than in the more caudal spaces. Within the same space, activation is greater dorsally and less ventrally [20, 21]. These differential patterns of activation are preserved even after all afferent feedback is removed by phrenic nerve section and complete thoracic rhizotomy, so the patterns appear to be "hard-wired" (studies made in dogs) [22, 23].

Neuromuscular Respiratory Failure

Causes of Neuromuscular Respiratory Failure

In the patient with neuromuscular disease, there are different factors that can contribute to the development of respiratory failure [24].

- Upper airway problems: weakness of facial, oropharyngeal, laryngeal muscles interfere with swallowing and secretion clearance, increasing risk of aspiration. There is also the potential for upper airway obstruction, especially when the patient is in a supine position.
- Inspiratory muscle weakness leads to poor lung expansion which causes microatelectasis, with resultant ventilation/perfusion mismatch and then hypoxemia.
- Small tidal volumes secondary to tachypnea cause more atelectasis.
- Expiratory muscle weakness causes inefficient cough and secretion clearance, increasing the risk of aspiration and pneumonia.
- Other complications such as pneumonia or pulmonary embolus can also exacerbate the ventilatory demand on an already weakened patient.

Clinical Presentation and Evaluation of Patients with Neuromuscular Respiratory Failure

The initial evaluation of a patient with neuromuscular respiratory failure should include (as in patient with other conditions) a detailed history and physical exam; especially looking for clues or signs of cardiac, pulmonary, infectious etiologies of respiratory problems. Regarding neuromuscular conditions, questioning the patient and family about time of onset and progression of weakness, concurrent fatigue, diplopia, dysphagia, weight loss, voice changes, the site of onset, and symmetry (or asymmetry) and progression of presentation can also provide clues towards the etiology. For example, a slowly progressive, initially asymmetric pure motor problem suggests a motor neuron problem such as amyotrophic lateral sclerosis. A rapid onset, ascending weakness and numbness with eventual generalization and areflexia, suggests Guillain-Barré syndrome. A patient with asymmetric intermittent diplopia, eyelid ptosis, dysphagia, and fatigability is more consistent with myasthenia gravis.

Patients with neuromuscular respiratory failure can complain of shortness of breath or dyspnea. This is typically worse when lying supine (orthopnea) or when immerse in water up to the chest (because the water pushes against the abdomen, increasing the intra-abdominal pressure and as a result the diaphragm moves upwards into the thoracic cavity, reducing its size, and the tidal volume).

Patients that have developed respiratory failure very slowly may deny dyspnea because they are already limited physically, are mostly sedentary, and do not exercise. In those cases, the presence of certain symptoms can suggest nocturnal hypoventilation: nonrefreshing sleep, early morning somnolence, morning headaches, day-time fatigue.

Symptoms of facial and oral weakness include diplopia and eyelid ptosis (fatigable or non-fatigable), dysphagia, drooling, nasal voice, and choking [11, 25].

In the physical exam, it is important to look for signs of impending catastrophic respiratory failure or need for mechanical ventilation, as identification of those signs indicates the need to transfer the patient to an intensive care unit and start ventilatory support. Absolute criteria for intubation include impaired consciousness, cardiac or respiratory arrest, arrhythmias, blood-gas alterations, and bulbar dysfunction with aspiration.

In patients without those absolute criteria, regular monitoring for other signs can be helpful to decide about monitoring or intubation [24–26]:

– Rapid shallow breathing
– Accessory muscle use (palpation is more helpful than observation)
– Paradoxical breathing (inward abdominal movement during inspiration)
– Orthopnea
– Cough after swallowing (aspiration)
– Diaphoresis
– Tachycardia
– Staccato speech (the need to pause between words while speaking)
– Trapezius and neck muscle weakness (which correlates with diaphragm weakness)
– Single breath count test; patient counts out loud after a maximal inspiration; normal count is 30–50; a single breath count <20 indicates very reduced vital capacity (approximately 100 mL per each number)

Regarding paradoxical breathing, when the diaphragm is paralyzed, the ribcage expansion is performed mostly by the accessory inspiratory muscles. With ribcage expansion, the intrapleural pressure drops and the flaccid diaphragm moves upwards inside the chest and the abdominal wall moves passively inwards during inspiration causing "paradoxical abdominal movement" or paradoxical breathing (it is called paradoxical because the abdomen is supposed to move outwards during normal inspiration). This paradoxical movement is more marked in a supine position and the abdominal movement towards the thorax decreases the tidal volume. When the person is in a standing position, gravity partially counteracts the upward motion of the abdominal contents and improves tidal volume during inspiration. For this reason, patients with diaphragmatic weakness have worsening of their symptoms when lying flat on their backs and have smaller supine than standing vital capacity. Weakness also worsens when immersed in water up to the chest level. The symptoms can also worsen at night because the majority of neural drive to the respiratory muscles during sleep is directed to the diaphragm which in this case is weak [26].

When the intercostal and abdominal muscles are weak and the diaphragm is intact, patients have paradoxical ribcage movement. When the diaphragm lowers the intrapleural pressure during inspiration, the intercostal spaces and the upper ribcage move inwards due to the flaccid intercostal muscle tone. When the patient stands up, the abdominal contents fall and the abdominal wall bulges out due its flaccid tone. This causes the diaphragm to be flattened and infective for inspiration. In these cases, patients may experience shortness of breath in the upright position [26].

The physical examination should also include testing of muscle strength in face, oropharyngeal area and extremities, checking for fatigability, and observation of extraocular movements, sensory loss or sensory level, coordination, reflexes, cardiac and lung auscultation, abdominal exam, and observing for fasciculations (including facial and tongue muscles).

Laboratory Assessment of Patients with Neuromuscular Respiratory Failure

As mentioned before, weakness of inspiratory muscles will reduce tidal volume causing atelectasis and consequent arterial hypoxemia [27]. When weakness starts slowly, this can be unrecognized and present initially only at night during REM sleep (due to decreased respiratory drive and hypotonia of respiratory muscles other than the diaphragm during REM). For this reason, nocturnal pulse oximetry is very helpful in diagnosing these cases. It is important to remember that hypercapnia is a late feature in this form of respiratory failure and usually heralds impending respiratory arrest.

Patients that are admitted should have periodic (every 4–6 h) assessment of bedside respiratory function by spirometry including forced vital capacity (FVC), maximal inspiratory pressure (MIP) also called negative-inspiratory force (NIF), and maximal expiratory pressure (MEP). They should also have an arterial blood gas and a chest X-ray.

It is important to remember that these spirometry tests are effort dependent, so the patient needs to give maximal effort during testing. Another potential caveat is that facial weakness prevents adequate mouth sealing around the spirometer which will cause air leak and falsely low values. This problem can be avoided with the use of a mask device.

A normal VC is 60–70 mL/kg. When VC is <30 mL/kg, the patient develops weak cough and atelectasis and a VC <15 mL/kg is an absolute criterion for intubation. A MEP <40 cm H_2O (normal 100 cm H_2O in adults) is associated with the inability to cough and clear secretions. A MIP > −20 cm H_2O (normal < −80 cm H_2O in male, <−70 cm H_2O in female) precludes effective ventilation [24, 26]. There is a thought that static respiratory pressures (MIP and MEP) are more sensitive than VC in the detection of respiratory muscles weakness [28].

Values of FVC and MIP are higher when the patients are in the standing or leaning forward positions and lower when they are supine. For this reason, it is also important to measure FVC, and MIP in the standing and supine position. A drop of >20% from upright to supine positions suggests diaphragmatic weakness [25, 29, 30]. It is also important to look for major discrepancies in values of FVC, MIP, and MEP, which can suggest technical errors in measurement; however, patients with myasthenia gravis can have fluctuating values which reflects the fluctuating (fatigable) nature of their disease. A normal FVC with no significant fall when moving to a supine position indicates that neuromuscular weakness is unlikely to be the cause for the respiratory symptoms. However, as mentioned before myasthenia gravis weakness can fluctuate significantly [11, 24, 25].

A more accurate measurement of diaphragmatic strength is obtained by measuring transdiaphragmatic pressure (Pdi); however, this test is not done routinely because it is an invasive test. When sniff Pdi falls below 30 cm H_2O, abdominal paradox develops [31]. This correlates with severe orthopnea and abdominal paradox occurring only when the strength of the diaphragm has been reduced to 25% of normal [32].

Peak cough flow can be measured at bedside with a peak flow meter. The normal range in adults is 360–840 L/min. A value <160–200 L/min may be associated with the inability to clear secretions and indicates that assisted coughing may be needed [25].

Another important point to remember is that arterial blood gases become abnormal late in the course of neuromuscular respiratory failure. Patients with established neuromuscular respiratory failure will show hypoxemia and compensated respiratory acidosis (elevated $PaCO_2$ and bicarbonate with normal or mildly reduced pH). If the pH and bicarbonate are elevated with normal PaO_2 and $PaCO_2$, it indicates nocturnal hypoventilation [24, 25]. Hypercapnia will not usually develop until respiratory muscle strength (measured as average of MIP and MEP) is reduced to <30% of normal [33].

A routine chest X-ray should be performed in all patients with neuromuscular respiratory failure, as it provides information about cardiac silhouette, possible consolidations, pneumonia, atelectasis, scoliosis, or unilateral diaphragmatic paralysis (suggested by a raised hemidiaphragm) [25].

Other tests need to be ordered to investigate the cause of the neuromuscular weakness. These orders should be based on the clinical history, physical exam findings, and potential differential diagnosis. They include nerve conduction studies (NCS) and electromyography (EMG) with possible repetitive nerve stimulation and diaphragm testing, blood/serum electrolytes, myasthenia antibodies, creatine kinase,

Table 2.1 Causes of neuromuscular respiratory failure according to nervous system site of injury (list is not all-inclusive)

Motor neuron	Motor neuron disease (amyotrophic lateral sclerosis, spinal muscular atrophy, Kennedy's disease, etc.)
	Poliomyelitis
	Postpolio syndrome
	West Nile virus and other viruses
Nerve root and peripheral nerve	Guillain-Barré syndrome
	Critical illness polyneuropathy
	Acute onset of chronic inflammatory demyelinating polyneuropathy (CIDP)
	Porphyria
	Arsenic, thallium poisoning
	Diphtheritic polyneuropathy
	Phrenic neuropathy
	Vasculitis
	Toxins: tetrodotoxin, etc.
	Some Charcot Marie Tooth neuropathy types
Neuromuscular junction	Myasthenia gravis
	Lambert-Eaton myasthenic syndrome
	Botulism
	Organophosphate poisoning
	Tick paralysis
	Other toxins: Snake, scorpion, spider venom
	Hypermagnesemia
Muscle	Critical illness myopathy
	Acid–maltase deficiency
	Hyperthyroidism
	Hypophosphatemia
	Hypokalemia
	Muscular dystrophy
	Mitochondrial myopathy
	Rhabdomyolysis
	Inflammatory myopathy
	Toxins: Barium

aldolase, voltage-gated calcium channel antibodies, antiganglioside antibodies, lumbar puncture, nerve and muscle biopsy and should be based on clinical suspicion. Table 2.1 lists the most common causes of neuromuscular respiratory failure.

Predictors of the Need for Mechanical Ventilation in Patients with Neuromuscular Respiratory Failure

It is very important to identify those patients that will develop worsening respiratory failure and will require some type of ventilator support, in order to prevent the complications of emergent intubation.

When to Intubate and Start Mechanical Ventilation (Table 2.2)

Most of the studies performed to identify predictors of the need for mechanical ventilation (MV) have focused on Guillain-Barré syndrome but their results can be extrapolated to other neuromuscular diagnosis (with the caveat that conditions such as myasthenia gravis can present variable results that correlate with fluctuating muscle strength testing).

When to Intubate and Start Mechanical Ventilation (Table 2.2)

As mentioned before, absolute criteria for intubation include impaired consciousness, cardiac or respiratory arrest, arrhythmias, blood-gas alterations, and bulbar dysfunction with aspiration. In addition, patients with the following features will benefit from early ventilator support: patients with the 20/30/40 rule (VC < 20 mL/kg; MIP > −30 cm H_2O; MEP < 40 cm H_2O); reduction in VC, MIP, or MEP > 30%; hypoxemia PO_2 <70 mmHg on room air, PCO_2 > 50 mmHg with acidosis; dysarthria, dysphagia, and impaired gag reflex.

Predictors of MV in GBS

In 2001, Lawn et al. reported a retrospective study in patients with GBS admitted to an intensive care unit to identify clinical features associated with progression to

Table 2.2 History and exam findings indicative of respiratory failure and possible need for intubation

Signs and symptoms concerning for impeding respiratory failure and need for intubation or ventilator support	Dysphagia
	Dysphonia
	Dyspnea at rest or on exertion
	Diaphoresis
	Stridor
	Shallow breathing
	Tachycardia
	Staccato speech
	Accessory respiratory muscle use (visible or palpable)
	Orthopnea
	Cough after swallowing
	Paradoxical breathing
	Weak cough
Signs and symptoms of chronic neuromuscular respiratory failure	Morning headaches
	Excessive day-time sleepiness
	Lack of restful sleep
Objective findings concerning for impeding respiratory failure and need for intubation or ventilator support	Breath count <20
	FVC < 20 mL/kg
	MIP (NIF) > −30 cm H_2O
	MEP < 40 cm H_2O
	Drop > 30% in FVC, MIP, or MEP
	Nocturnal desaturation
	Hypoxemia
	Hypercapnia

respiratory failure in 60 patients that received mechanical ventilation vs. 54 patients that did not need it. Progression to mechanical ventilation was more likely to occur in patients with rapid disease progression (<7 days), bulbar dysfunction, bilateral facial weakness, or dysautonomia. A vital capacity <20 mL/kg, MIP > −30 cm H_2O, and MEP < 40 cm H_2O (20/30/40 rule) or a reduction of >30% in FVC, MIP, or MEP also correlated with need for mechanical ventilation [34].

In 2006, Durand et al. published a prospective study in 154 patients with GBS, of which 34 (22%) required mechanical ventilation. The risk of respiratory failure was greater in patients with demyelinating GBS (85% vs. 51%). A vital capacity <81% of normal and a proximal/distal compound muscle action potential (p/d CMAP) ratio of the common peroneal nerve (CPN) <55.6% were also associated with higher risk of mechanical ventilation (Odds ratio (OR) of 29.3–41 for patients with <55.6% p/d CMAP; and of 16.1–17.1 for patients with >55.6% p/d CPN CMAP and VC <81% (OR values in fitting and validation sets, respectively)) [35].

In 2003, Sharshar et al. reported on the same topic on their study of patients with GBS enrolled in two multicenter randomized trials of plasma exchange. They included 722 patients, of which 313 (43%) required mechanical ventilation. The predictors for endotracheal mechanical ventilation were time from onset of motor symptoms to admission <7 days (OR 2.51), inability to cough (OR 2.53), inability to stand (OR 2.53), inability to lift the elbows off the bed (OR 2.99), inability to lift the head (OR 2.99), and liver enzyme elevation (OR 2.09). There was no clear explanation for the relationship between elevated liver enzymes and need for mechanical ventilation. When only the 196 patients that have their vital capacity measured were analyzed, time from onset of motor symptoms to admission <7 days (OR 5.0), inability to lift the head (OR 5.0) and vital capacity <60% (OR 2.86) predicted mechanical ventilation. When these six risk factors were taken together, mechanical ventilation was required in 5% of 65 patients with zero predictors; 33% of 183 patients with 1 predictor; 71% of 205 patients with two predictors; 84% of 136 patients with 3 predictors; 69% of patients with four predictors; 42% of 43 patients with five predictors; and 100% of 9 patients with six predictors [36].

The importance of phrenic motor latency and/or amplitude and its correlation with the need of mechanical ventilation has not been clear with some studies finding it helpful [37] and others not better than clinical features and vital capacity [38].

In 2010, Walgaard et al. published a study on 397 GBS patients that was then validated in 191 patients more. Of those patients, 22% in the first and 14% in the validation cohorts required mechanical ventilation within the first week after admission. The number of days between onset of weakness and admission, Medical Research Council sum score (MRC sum score, defined as the sum of MRC scores of six different muscles measure bilaterally; ranging from 0 to 60) and the presence of facial and/or bulbar weakness were the main predictors of MV. They proposed the EGRIS (Erasmus GBS Respiratory Insufficiency Score) to predict the need for MV. The categories included in the score were: (1) days between onset of weakness and hospital admission (>7 days, 4–7 days, and ≤3 days for scores of 0, 1, and 2, respectively); (2) Facial and/or bulbar weakness at hospital admission (absent or present, scored 0 and 1, respectively); and MRC sum score at hospital admission (60–51, 50–41, 40–31, 30–21, and ≤20 for scores of 1, 2, 3, and 4, respectively). The total score could range from 0 to 7. When divided by risk, patients in a low, intermediate, and high EGRIS risk groups (0–2, 3–4, and 5–7 total scores) have 4%, 24%, and 65% probability of respiratory insufficiency within the first week of admission [39].

Wu et al. published in 2015 a study done in 541 GBS patients of which 80 (14.8%) required MV. Multivariate analysis showed that shorter interval from onset to admission (average 3.5 vs. 6.3 days), facial nerve palsy, glossopharyngeal and vagal nerve deficits, and lower MRC sum score at nadir (16.6 vs. 41) were risk factors for MV [40].

Fourrier et al. studied 61 patients with GBS admitted to an ICU of which 40 (66%) required MV. When compared with those that did not require MV, the MV patients were more likely to have cardiovascular autonomic dysfunction (OR 10.66) or were unable to lift their head above the bed (OR 9.86). Cardiovascular autonomic dysfunction was defined as an increase or decrease of 40 mmHg in systolic blood pressure, spontaneous or induced bradycardia, decrease in heart rate of >20 beats per minutes; or spontaneous tachycardia with 23 heart rate >120 beats per minute without fever [41].

Orlikowski et al. found that in 16 GBS patients admitted to the ICU, severity of tongue weakness correlated with need for mechanical ventilation [42].

In 138 patients with GBS, of which 53 required MV, Paul et al. identified simultaneous motor weakness in upper and lower extremities, upper extremity strength <3/5 at nadir, and the presence of bulbar weakness as risk factors associated with the need for mechanical ventilation. Preservation of deep tendon reflexes in upper extremities was associated with a decreased need for MV [43].

A small study of 55 patients with GBS of which 28 (50.9%) needed MV identified bulbar weakness and time to peak limb weakness ≤5 days as predictors for respiratory insufficiency [44].

In 46 patients with GBS of which 28 required mechanical ventilation, identified early peak disability (33 h vs. 6 days), bulbar dysfunction, and autonomic instability as independent predictors of MV [45].

Table 2.3 lists the risk factors associated with the need for MV in GBS patients identified in the different studies.

Although about 30% of patients with GBS will eventually require MV, it is important to remember that endotracheal intubation in patients with GBS can trigger profound bradycardia and blood pressure changes and even cause cardiac arrest. Depolarizing agents such as succinylcholine must be avoided due to the risk of fatal hyperkalemia due to increased chemosensitivity of denervated muscles [46]. Mechanical ventilation is also associated with worse outcome in GBS, and in some cases up to 20% mortality. Furthermore, patients with GBS and respiratory failure will likely not benefit from noninvasive ventilation, and this procedure can leave them exposed to the risk of emergent intubation [47].

Figure 2.1 shows a proposed algorithm to respiratory failure in patients with GBS.

Table 2.3 Predictors of the need for mechanical ventilation in patients with Guillain-Barré syndrome according to different studies

Predictors/study	Lawn 60 vs. 54	Durand 34 vs. 120	Paul 53 vs. 85	Sharshar 313 vs. 409	Walgaard 83 vs. 294	Wu 80 vs. 461	Fourrier 40 vs. 21	Toamad 28 vs. 27	Sundar 28 vs. 18
Rapid progression	<7 days							<5 days	33 h
Bulbar dysfunction	+	+	+	+	+			+	+
Bilateral facial weakness	+	+		+	+	+			
Dysautonomia	+			+			+		+
VC <20 MIP>−30 MEP <40	+								
Drop >30% VC, MEP, MIP	+								
p/d CMAP peroneal and VC <81%		+							
Demyelinating GBS		+							
3/5 MRC UE at peak			+						
Simultaneous UE and LE weakness			+						
Time from onset to admission <7 days				+	+	+			
Inability to stand				+					
Inability to lift elbow above bed				+					
Inability to lift head above bed		+		+			+		
Ineffective cough				+					
Liver enzyme elevation				+					
VC <60% on admission				+					
MRC score admission					+				
Glossopharyngeal and vagal nerve deficits						+			
Low MRC score at nadir (16.6)						+			

Each column corresponds to a different study on the predictors of mechanical ventilation (MV) in patients with Guillain-Barré syndrome. To get an idea of the study size, the numbers below the authors' names represents the number of patient that required (first number) vs. those that did not require (second number) MV in each study

VC vital capacity, *MIP* maximal inspiratory force, *MEP* maximal expiratory force, *p/d* proximal/distal ratio, *CMAP* compound muscle action potential, *MRC* Medical Research Council, *UE* upper extremity, *LE* lower extremity, *GBS* Guillain-Barré syndrome

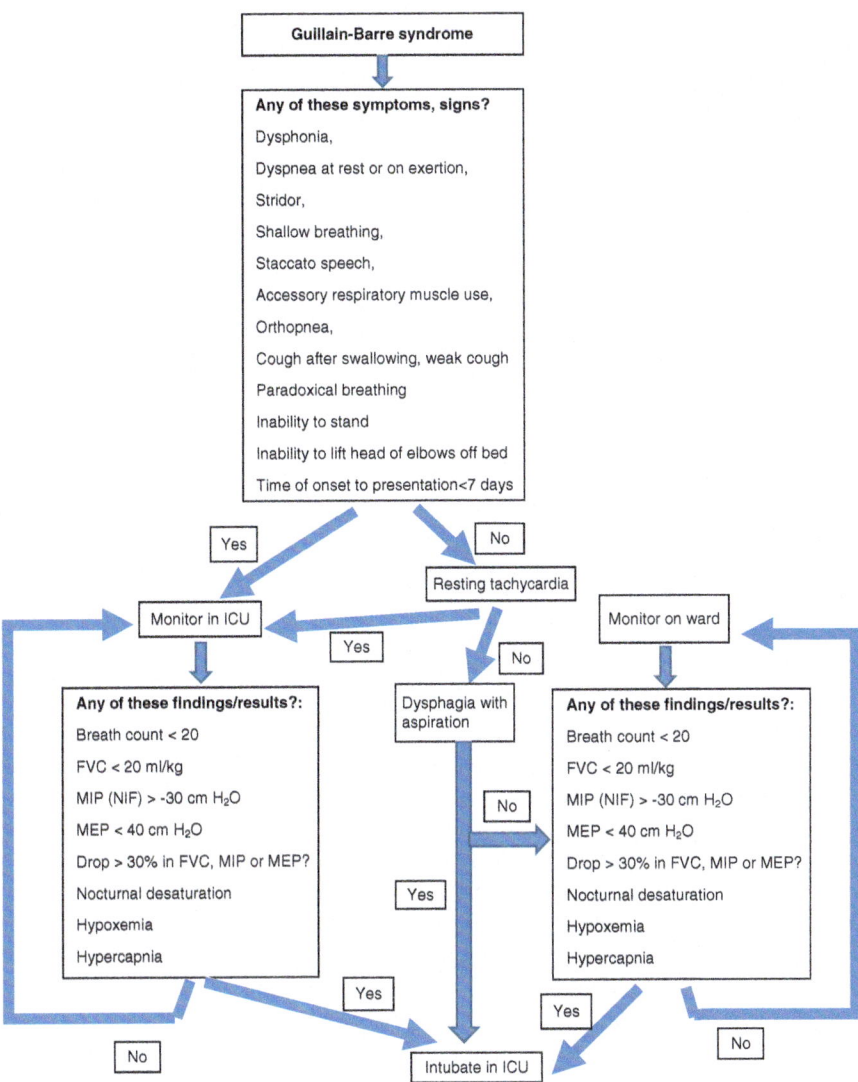

Fig. 2.1 Approach to respiratory failure in the patient with Guillain-Barré syndrome

Predictors of Prolonged Intubation in GBS

The duration of intubation in GBS patients usually ranges from 18 to 29 days. It is also important to predict which patients will require prolonged intubation so that tracheostomy and other care can be planned accordingly, and some studies have been done in that respect. Nguyen et al. found that in 44 intubated GBS patients, of which 14 (31.8%) were successfully extubated; a NIF <−50 cm H_2O and an increase of vital capacity value from pre-intubation to pre-extubation by >4 mL/kg on the extubation day were significantly associated with successful extubation [48]. In a

Table 2.4 Predictors of prolonged intubation in patients with Guillain-Barré syndrome

Study	Predictor
Nguyen (>2 weeks) 44 patients	MIP > −50 cm H_2O on extubation day Increment of VC < 4 mL/kg by extubation day
Lawn (>3 weeks) 37 patients	Pulmonary function score (PFS) (sum of FVC, MIP and MEP values) at day 12 post-intubation > day 1 post-intubation
Walgaard (>2 weeks) 150 patients	Inability to lift arms above the bed 1 week after intubation Axonal loss or inexcitable nerves 1 week after intubation
Lawn (>3 weeks) 60 patients	Older age Underlying pulmonary disease
Fourrier (>2 weeks) 61 patients	Lack of foot dorsiflexion and presence of sciatic nerve conduction block at the end of immunotherapy (days 8–10)

Time in parenthesis indicates definition of prolonged intubation in each study. Number of patients intubated is included for reference
VC vital capacity, *MIP* maximal inspiratory force, *MEP* maximal expiratory force

different study, Lawn et al. compared GBS patients with MV for <3 and >3 weeks (10 vs. 27 patients, respectively) and found that the pulmonary function score (PF score), defined as the sum of VC, MIP, and MEP values, was higher at 12 days after intubation vs. its value on the day of intubation (PFS ratio day 12/day 1 value >1). The sensitivity of PF ratio <1 for predicting duration of MV >3 weeks was 70%; the specificity and positive predictive value were 100%. The authors used values at day 12 because in their opinion, the decision to perform tracheostomy is made around that time [49]. In a study of 552 patients with GBS, of which 150 (27%) required mechanical ventilation; the predictors of prolonged MV (defined as duration ≥14 days) were the inability to lift arms from the bed (MRC 0–2) 1 week after intubation (87% vs. 69%) and axonal degeneration or unexcitable nerves on nerve conduction studies (100% vs. 75%) [50]. In other small study with only 60 patients with GBS, older age (average 63 vs. 47 years) and underlying pulmonary disease were associated with intubation >3 weeks [51]. In another study of 61 patients admitted to the ICU, of which 40 (66%) required MV; lack of foot dorsiflexion and the presence of sciatic nerve conduction block at the end of immunotherapy (8–10 days) were associated with prolonged MV (>15 days) [41]. The predictors of prolonged intubation in patients with Guillain-Barré syndrome are laid out in Table 2.4.

Predictors of MV in Myasthenia Gravis

Patients with myasthenia gravis can develop respiratory failure or myasthenic crisis requiring admission to an intensive care unit. Because of the fluctuating nature of their disease, patients with myasthenic crisis and incipient respiratory muscle fatigue or prominent muscle weakness need to be followed closely in an intensive care unit. This includes serial measurements of vital capacity and MIP every 4–6 h. The factors that predict MV in Guillain-Barré syndrome such as 20/30/40 rule, bulbar and facial weakness can also be used to decide to start ventilator support. An important difference between myasthenia gravis and GBS patients is that in some MG patients, noninvasive ventilation such as Bipap can avert intubation, so in some myasthenic patients a trial of Bipap before intubation can be helpful. Bipap averted intubation in 14/24 and 7/9 patients with myasthenic crisis in two different studies and was used for up to 15 days, including patients that presented with bulbar weakness [52, 53]. However, if MG patients are found to have hypercapnia in arterial blood gas testing, they will likely fail a trial of Bipap and those patients will need to be intubated instead. Other characteristics such as VC, MIP, MEP, or the presence of secretions did not predict Bipap failure. Patient should also be intubated if they have other pulmonary complications such as atelectasis, infiltrates or pneumonia, and preexisting lung disease. Patients that are successfully treated with Bipap have lower rates of pulmonary complications (atelectasis and pneumonia) than those that are intubated [52, 53].

Figure 2.2 shows a proposed approach to respiratory failure in patients with myasthenia gravis exacerbation.

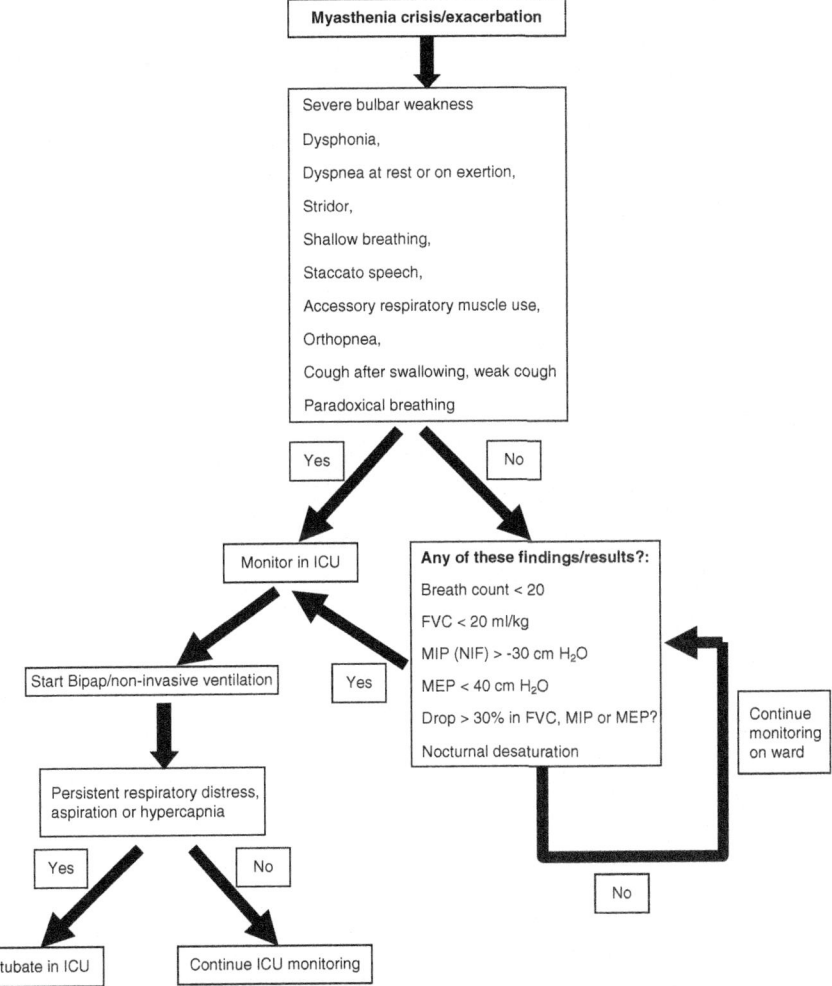

Fig. 2.2 Approach to respiratory failure in a patient with myasthenia exacerbation

Predictors of Prolonged Intubation in Myasthenia Gravis

Thomas reported on a study of 53 patients with myasthenic crisis of which 4% died. Among those patients, pre-intubation serum bicarbonate ≥30 mg/dL, peak vital capacity day 1–6 post-intubation <25 mL/kg and age >50 were independent predictors of prolonged intubation (>2 weeks). The proportion of patients intubated >2 weeks was 0% with no risk factors, 21% with one risk factor, 46% with two risk factors, and 88% with three risk factors [54].

Conclusion

Neuromuscular respiratory failure is an important condition that should be recognized early to avoid emergent intubation or catastrophic respiratory failure. A careful history and physical examination, with particular attention to clinical clues of respiratory distress and the use of other laboratory and pulmonary tests that predict the need of ventilatory support can aid in the diagnosis, treatment, and improve prognosis in this group of patients. Among the possible causes, GBS and MG are the most frequent, and both are treatable. This reinforces the need to be aware of their presentation. Careful monitoring of the bulbar and respiratory function is needed in this group of patients to maximize good outcome.

Key Points

1. The diaphragm is responsible for 60–70% of the tidal volume in normal breathing. Its muscle fibers radiate from a central tendon and can be divided into two portions: crural diaphragm and costal diaphragm.
2. Expiratory muscles include the internal intercostals, and the four abdominal muscles (rectus abdominis, external oblique, internal oblique, and transverse abdominis). At rest, expiration is mostly passive by recoil of the thoracic cage.
3. The pre-Botzinger complex located caudal to the rVRG in the medulla is the central respiratory rhythm generator. The inspiratory muscles are activated using neuromechanical matching, in which neural drive is higher to the muscles with the greatest mechanical advantage for inspiration.
4. The 20/30/40 rule (VC <20 mL/kg, MIP>−30 cm H_2O, MEP <40 cm H_2O) indicates the need of mechanical ventilation in patients with neuromuscular respiratory failure.
5. In neuromuscular disorders, symptoms of facial and oral weakness include diplopia and eyelid ptosis (fatigable or non-fatigable), dysphagia, drooling, nasal voice, and choking.
6. Neuromuscular conditions that absolutely require intubation include impaired consciousness, cardiac or respiratory arrest, arrhythmias, blood-gas alterations, and bulbar dysfunction with aspiration.
7. A normal vital capacity (VC) is 60–70 mL/kg. When VC is <30 mL/kg, the patient develops weak cough and atelectasis and a VC <15 mL/kg is an absolute criterion for intubation.

8. Arterial blood gases become abnormal late in the course of neuromuscular respiratory failure. Patients with established neuromuscular respiratory failure will show hypoxemia and compensated respiratory acidosis.
9. Because of the fluctuating nature of their disease, patients with myasthenic crisis and incipient respiratory muscle fatigue or prominent muscle weakness need to be followed closely in an intensive care unit.
10. Inability to stand, or lift the head and elbows off the bed can predict the need for mechanical ventilation in GBS patients.
11. Noninvasive ventilation such as Bipap can prevent intubation in patients with myasthenia gravis, except in those with hypercapnia in arterial blood gas testing.
12. In GBS patients, the pulmonary function score (PFS) (sum of VC, MIP, and MEP) at day 12 vs. day 1 after intubation can predict duration of intubation >3 weeks.
13. In myasthenia crisis patients, pre-intubation serum bicarbonate ≥30 mg/dL, peak vital capacity at day 1–6 post-intubation <25 mL/kg and age >50 can be used to predict duration of intubation longer than 2 weeks.

References

1. Ratnovsky A, Elad D, Halpern P. Mechanics of respiratory muscles. Respir Physiol Neurobiol. 2008;163(1–3):82–9.
2. Caruso P, Albuquerque AL, Santana PV, Cardenas LZ, Ferreira JG, Prina E, et al. Diagnostic methods to assess inspiratory and expiratory muscle strength. J Bras Pneumol. 2015;41(2):110–23.
3. Celli BR. Respiratory muscle function. Clin Chest Med. 1986;7(4):567–84.
4. Sieck GC. Physiological effects of diaphragm muscle denervation and disuse. Clin Chest Med. 1994;15(4):641–59.
5. Mantilla CB, Sieck GC. Phrenic motor unit recruitment during ventilatory and non-ventilatory behaviors. Respir Physiol Neurobiol. 2011;179(1):57–63.
6. Mantilla CB, Seven YB, Zhan WZ, Sieck GC. Diaphragm motor unit recruitment in rats. Respir Physiol Neurobiol. 2010;173(1):101–6.
7. Mantilla CB, Seven YB, Sieck GC. Convergence of pattern generator outputs on a common mechanism of diaphragm motor unit recruitment. Prog Brain Res. 2014;209:309–29.
8. De Troyer A, Kirkwood PA, Wilson TA. Respiratory action of the intercostal muscles. Physiol Rev. 2005;85(2):717–56.
9. De Troyer A, Estenne M. Coordination between rib cage muscles and diaphragm during quiet breathing in humans. J Appl Physiol Respir Environ Exerc Physiol. 1984;57(3):899–906.
10. De Troyer A, Sampson MG. Activation of the parasternal intercostals during breathing efforts in human subjects. J Appl Physiol Respir Environ Exerc Physiol. 1982;52(3):524–9.
11. Rabinstein AA. Acute neuromuscular respiratory failure. Continuum. 2015;21(5 Neurocritical Care):1324–45.
12. Wilson TA, Legrand A, Gevenois PA, De Troyer A. Respiratory effects of the external and internal intercostal muscles in humans. J Physiol. 2001;530(Pt 2):319–30.
13. Roussos C. Function and fatigue of respiratory muscles. Chest. 1985;88(2 Suppl):124S–32S.
14. Butler JE, Hudson AL, Gandevia SC. The neural control of human inspiratory muscles. Prog Brain Res. 2014;209:295–308.
15. Lee KZ, Fuller DD. Neural control of phrenic motoneuron discharge. Respir Physiol Neurobiol. 2011;179(1):71–9.

16. McCrimmon DR, Ramirez JM, Alford S, Zuperku EJ. Unraveling the mechanism for respiratory rhythm generation. Bioessays. 2000;22(1):6–9.
17. Feldman JL, Del Negro CA. Looking for inspiration: new perspectives on respiratory rhythm. Nat Rev Neurosci. 2006;7(3):232–42.
18. Tian GF, Peever JH, Duffin J. Bötzinger-complex expiratory neurons monosynaptically inhibit phrenic motoneurons in the decerebrate rat. Exp Brain Res. 1998;122(2):149–56.
19. Tian GF, Peever JH, Duffin J. Bötzinger-complex, bulbospinal expiratory neurones monosynaptically inhibit ventral-group respiratory neurones in the decerebrate rat. Exp Brain Res. 1999;124(2):173–80.
20. Butler JE, Gandevia SC. The output from human inspiratory motoneurone pools. J Physiol. 2008;586(5):1257–64.
21. Butler JE. Drive to the human respiratory muscles. Respir Physiol Neurobiol. 2007;159(2):115–26.
22. De Troyer A, Legrand A. Inhomogeneous activation of the parasternal intercostals during breathing. J Appl Physiol (1985). 1995;79(1):55–62.
23. Hudson AL, Gandevia SC, Butler JE. Control of human inspiratory motoneurones during voluntary and involuntary contractions. Respir Physiol Neurobiol. 2011;179(1):23–33.
24. Mehta S. Neuromuscular disease causing acute respiratory failure. Respir Care. 2006;51(9):1016–21; discussion 1021–3
25. Hutchinson D, Whyte K. Neuromuscular disease and respiratory failure. Pract Neurol. 2008;8(4):229–37.
26. Hughes RA, Bihari D. Acute neuromuscular respiratory paralysis. J Neurol Neurosurg Psychiatry. 1993;56(4):334–43.
27. Kelly BJ, Luce JM. The diagnosis and management of neuromuscular diseases causing respiratory failure. Chest. 1991;99(6):1485–94.
28. Black LF, Hyatt RE. Maximal static respiratory pressures in generalized neuromuscular disease. Am Rev Respir Dis. 1971;103(5):641–50.
29. Vilke GM, Chan TC, Neuman T, Clausen JL. Spirometry in normal subjects in sitting, prone, and supine positions. Respir Care. 2000;45(4):407–10.
30. Allen SM, Hunt B, Green M. Fall in vital capacity with posture. Br J Dis Chest. 1985;79(3):267–71.
31. Mier-Jedrzejowicz A, Brophy C, Moxham J, Green M. Assessment of diaphragm weakness. Am Rev Respir Dis. 1988;137(4):877–83.
32. Syabbalo N. Assessment of respiratory muscle function and strength. Postgrad Med J. 1998;74(870):208–15.
33. Braun NM, Arora NS, Rochester DF. Respiratory muscle and pulmonary function in polymyositis and other proximal myopathies. Thorax. 1983;38(8):616–23.
34. Lawn ND, Fletcher DD, Henderson RD, Wolter TD, Wijdicks EF. Anticipating mechanical ventilation in Guillain-Barré syndrome. Arch Neurol. 2001;58(6):893–8.
35. Durand MC, Porcher R, Orlikowski D, Aboab J, Devaux C, Clair B, et al. Clinical and electrophysiological predictors of respiratory failure in Guillain-Barré syndrome: a prospective study. Lancet Neurol. 2006;5(12):1021–8.
36. Sharshar T, Chevret S, Bourdain F, Raphaël JC, French Cooperative Group on Plasma Exchange in Guillain-Barré Syndrome. Early predictors of mechanical ventilation in Guillain-Barré syndrome. Crit Care Med. 2003;31(1):278–83.
37. Ito H, Fujita K, Kinoshita Y, Takanashi Y, Kusaka H. Phrenic nerve conduction in the early stage of Guillain-Barre syndrome might predict the respiratory failure. Acta Neurol Scand. 2007;116(4):255–8.
38. Durand MC, Prigent H, Sivadon-Tardy V, Orlikowski D, Caudie C, Devaux C, et al. Significance of phrenic nerve electrophysiological abnormalities in Guillain-Barré syndrome. Neurology. 2005;65(10):1646–9.
39. Walgaard C, Lingsma HF, Ruts L, Drenthen J, van Koningsveld R, Garssen MJ, et al. Prediction of respiratory insufficiency in Guillain-Barré syndrome. Ann Neurol. 2010;67(6):781–7.

40. Wu X, Li C, Zhang B, Shen D, Li T, Liu K, et al. Predictors for mechanical ventilation and short-term prognosis in patients with Guillain-Barré syndrome. Crit Care. 2015;19:310.
41. Fourrier F, Robriquet L, Hurtevent JF, Spagnolo S. A simple functional marker to predict the need for prolonged mechanical ventilation in patients with Guillain-Barré syndrome. Crit Care. 2011;15(1):R65.
42. Orlikowski D, Terzi N, Blumen M, Sharshar T, Raphael JC, Annane D, et al. Tongue weakness is associated with respiratory failure in patients with severe Guillain-Barré syndrome. Acta Neurol Scand. 2009;119(6):364–70.
43. Paul BS, Bhatia R, Prasad K, Padma MV, Tripathi M, Singh MB. Clinical predictors of mechanical ventilation in Guillain-Barré syndrome. Neurol India. 2012;60(2):150–3.
44. Toamad U, Kongkamol C, Setthawatcharawanich S, Limapichat K, Phabphal K, Sathirapanya P. Clinical presentations as predictors of prolonged mechanical ventilation in Guillain-Barré syndrome in an institution with limited medical resources. Singapore Med J. 2015;56(10):558–61.
45. Sundar U, Abraham E, Gharat A, Yeolekar ME, Trivedi T, Dwivedi N. Neuromuscular respiratory failure in Guillain-Barre Syndrome: evaluation of clinical and electrodiagnostic predictors. J Assoc Physicians India. 2005;53:764–8.
46. Orlikowski D, Prigent H, Sharshar T, Lofaso F, Raphael JC. Respiratory dysfunction in Guillain-Barré syndrome. Neurocrit Care. 2004;1(4):415–22.
47. Wijdicks EF, Roy TK. BiPAP in early Guillain-Barré syndrome may fail. Can J Neurol Sci. 2006;33(1):105–6.
48. Nguyen TN, Badjatia N, Malhotra A, Gibbons FK, Qureshi MM, Greenberg SA. Factors predicting extubation success in patients with Guillain-Barré syndrome. Neurocrit Care. 2006;5(3):230–4.
49. Lawn ND, Wijdicks EF. Post-intubation pulmonary function test in Guillain-Barré syndrome. Muscle Nerve. 2000;23(4):613–6.
50. Walgaard C, Lingsma HF, van Doorn PA, van der Jagt M, Steyerberg EW, Jacobs BC. Tracheostomy or not: prediction of prolonged mechanical ventilation in Guillain-Barré syndrome. Neurocrit Care. 2017;26:6–13.
51. Lawn ND, Wijdicks EF. Tracheostomy in Guillain-Barré syndrome. Muscle Nerve. 1999;22(8):1058–62.
52. Rabinstein A, Wijdicks EF. BiPAP in acute respiratory failure due to myasthenic crisis may prevent intubation. Neurology. 2002;59(10):1647–9.
53. Seneviratne J, Mandrekar J, Wijdicks EF, Rabinstein AA. Noninvasive ventilation in myasthenic crisis. Arch Neurol. 2008;65(1):54–8.
54. Thomas CE, Mayer SA, Gungor Y, Swarup R, Webster EA, Chang I, et al. Myasthenic crisis: clinical features, mortality, complications, and risk factors for prolonged intubation. Neurology. 1997;48(5):1253–60.

Suggested Reading

Butler JE, Hudson AL, Gandevia SC. The neural control of human inspiratory muscles. Prog Brain Res. 2014;209:295–308. (This paper describes the principle of neuromechanical matching in which neural drive is higher in the muscles with greatest mechanical advantage for inspiration to minimize metabolic costs).
Durand MC, Porcher R, Orlikowski D, Aboab J, Devaux C, Clair B, et al. Clinical and electrophysiological predictors of respiratory failure in Guillain-Barré syndrome: a prospective study. Lancet Neurol. 2006;5(12):1021–8. (In this study done in 154 patients with GBS found that proximal/distal peroneal CMAP ratio and vital capacity <81% predicted need of mechanical ventilation).
Lawn ND, Wijdicks EF. Post-intubation pulmonary function test in Guillain-Barré syndrome. Muscle Nerve. 2000;23(4):613–6. (In this study in 37 GBS patient on mechanical ventilation,

the authors proposed the use of the PFS (Pulmonary Function Score) at day 12 to predict a duration of mechanical ventilation greater than 3 weeks).

Lawn ND, Fletcher DD, Henderson RD, Wolter TD, Wijdicks EF. Anticipating mechanical ventilation in Guillain-Barré syndrome. Arch Neurol. 2001;58(6):893–8. (Landmark paper in 114 GBS patients. It studied clinical and respiratory features associated with progression to mechanical ventilation in patients with GBS and proposed the now used 20/30/40 rule: VC<20 mL.kg, PImax<30 cmH$_2$O and PEmax <40 cmH$_2$O).

Rabinstein AA. Acute neuromuscular respiratory failure. Continuum. 2015;21(5 Neurocritical Care):1324–45. (Review of common causes, symptoms, and signs of acute neuromuscular respiratory failure, including Guillain-Barré syndrome and myasthenia gravis exacerbation).

Ratnovsky A, Elad D, Halpern P. Mechanics of respiratory muscles. Respir Physiol Neurobiol. 2008;163(1–3):82–9. (This paper provides a brief description of the the inspiratory and expiratory muscles and their main function).

Seneviratne J, Mandrekar J, Wijdicks EF, Rabinstein AA. Noninvasive ventilation in myasthenic crisis. Arch Neurol. 2008;65(1):54–8. (In this retrospective study in 60 patients with myasthenic crisis, the authors describe the usefulness of Bipap to prevent intubation, except in cases with hypercapnia in the arterial blood gas).

Sharshar T, Chevret S, Bourdain F, Raphaël JC, French Cooperative Group on Plasma Exchange in Guillain-Barré Syndrome. Early predictors of mechanical ventilation in Guillain-Barré syndrome. Crit Care Med. 2003;31(1):278–83. (In this study in 722 patients with GBS, the authors found useful clinical features that can predict the need for mechanical ventilation such as: time of onset to admission <7 days, inability to cough, inability to stand, inability to lift elbows or head, liver enzyme elevation, and vital capacity <60%).

Thomas CE, Mayer SA, Gungor Y, Swarup R, Webster EA, Chang I, et al. Myasthenic crisis: clinical features, mortality, complications, and risk factors for prolonged intubation. Neurology. 1997;48(5):1253–60. (Retrospective study in 53 patients with myasthenic crisis. The authors found that pre-intubation serum bicarbonate ≥30 mg/dl, peak vital capacity at day 1–6 post-intubation <25 mL/kg and age >50 can be used to predict duration of intubation longer than 2 weeks).

Walgaard C, Lingsma HF, Ruts L, Drenthen J, van Koningsveld R, Garssen MJ, et al. Prediction of respiratory insufficiency in Guillain-Barré syndrome. Ann Neurol. 2010;67(6):781–7. (Using a derivation and validation cohorts of 397 and 191 patients, respectively, this study proposed the EGRIS: Erasmus GBS Respiratory Insufficiency Score to predict the need for mechanical ventilation in patients with GBS).

Sleep Issues in Motor Neuron Diseases

3

Sushma Yerram, Pradeep C. Bollu, and Pradeep Sahota

Abbreviations

AHI	Apnea hypopnea index
ALS	Amyotrophic lateral sclerosis
LOSMoN	Late onset spinal motor neuronopathy
MA	Monomelic amyotrophy
NIV	Noninvasive ventilation
NREM	Non-rapid eye movement
OSA	Obstructive sleep apnea
PLMS	Periodic leg movements in sleep
PLS	Primary lateral sclerosis
PMA	Progressive muscular atrophy
PSG	Polysomnogram
REM	Rapid eye movement
RERA	Respiratory effort-related arousals
RLS	Restless leg syndrome
SDB	Sleep disordered breathing
SMA	Spinal muscular atrophy
SMA-LED	SMA with lower extremity predominance
SMN	Survival motor neuron
SNIP	Sniff nasal inspiratory pressure
SPSMA	Scapuloperoneal SMA

S. Yerram, M.D.
Department of Neurology, University of Rochester, Rochester, NY, USA

P. C. Bollu, M.D. (✉) · P. Sahota, M.D., F.A.A.N.
Department of Neurology, University of Missouri, Columbia, MO, USA
e-mail: BolluP@health.missouri.edu; sahotap@health.missouri.edu

Motor Neuron Disorders

Introduction

Motor neuron disorders are a group of neurodegenerative diseases involving progressive loss of motor neurons. It can involve upper motor neurons or lower motor neurons or both. They can be hereditary or sporadic. Their onset is prenatal (Spinal muscular atrophy Type 0) or childhood (Spinal muscular atrophy Type 1, 2, 3, etc.) or in adults (amyotrophic lateral sclerosis, progressive muscular atrophy, primary lateral sclerosis, etc.).

They are classified based on their age at onset, type of motor neuron degeneration (upper motor/ and lower motor neuron) all of which differ in inheritance pattern, genetics, clinical features, and prognosis.

Motor Neuron Disorders of Childhood

Spinal Muscular Atrophy (SMA) (Lower Motor Neuron Disease)

These are a group of autosomal recessive (AR) disorders with loss of anterior horn cells in spinal cord and brain stem (lower motor neurons).

SMA is the second most common autosomal recessive disease after cystic fibrosis affecting children. Its incidence is 1 in 11,000 live births [1]. They are caused by mutations in the survival motor neuron gene (SMN1 gene) on chromosome 15 Q11. SMN protein is important in RNA processing in all cells and has a critical but unknown function in survival of motor neurons.

A brief overview of the SMN1 and SMN2 gene is presented below.

Normal individuals have two forms of SMN gene, the telomeric (SMN1) and the centromeric (SMN2) arranged tandemly. SMN1 produces a functional protein. SMN2 is identical to SMN1 except for variation in a base pair that excludes exon 7 from transcription, causing degradation of its product. However, this exclusion is not complete, so SMN2 encodes a small amount of functional protein.

SMA patients have homozygous deletions of exon 7 of SMN1. Individuals with loss of functioning SMN1 but multiple copies of SMN2 produce a small amount of SMN protein and have milder symptoms.

SMAs occur in different phenotypes based on the number of copies in SMN2 gene. As the SMN2 gene copies increase, the severity of SMA decreases.

They are classified into five types based on age at onset and the motor functions/motor milestones they achieve.

Common clinical features resulting from degeneration of anterior horn cells include motor delays, hypotonia, proximal muscle weakness, and occasionally finger tremor and tongue fasciculations [1]. Prognosis depends on the SMA severity and degree of respiratory involvement.

SMA Type 0
This is the most severe form of SMA. Onset is in utero, evidenced by reduced fetal movements. At birth infants are floppy, areflexic with facial diplegia. They present with respiratory difficulties at birth requiring mechanical ventilation. Survival is rare beyond 6 months.

SMA Type 1
Type 1 manifest before 6 months of age. Infants have decreased muscle tone, absent reflexes, with poor neck control and attain a frog leg posture when laid down (due to hypotonia and absent neck holding). They can never sit unassisted. They have intercostal muscle weakness with relative sparing of diaphragm producing a pattern of paradoxical breathing/belly breathing from bell-shaped chest. They develop respiratory failure before 2 years of life.

SMA Type 2
Onset of type 2 is between 6 and 18 months, they can never walk unassisted. They have progressive proximal leg weakness more than arms. On exam, they are also areflexic like other SMAs.

With age they develop orthopedic complications related to progressive scoliosis, joint contractures. Pulmonary complications like restrictive lung disease arise from intercostal muscle weakness and scoliosis.

The most common cause of death in infants and children with types 1 and 2 SMA is respiratory failure.

SMA Type 3
This is a mild form of childhood SMA. Children can walk unassisted, but at some point they may need wheel chair due to progressive proximal weakness of legs. They have fewer or no orthopedic and pulmonary complications compared to SMA Type 2. Life expectancy is similar to age-matched general population groups.

Adult Onset Motor Neuron Diseases

SMA Type 4
Onset is generally after 30 years, rarely between 20 and 30 years. They have very mild proximal leg weakness. They have no alteration of life expectancy from the disease.

SMA Syndromes
These are a subset of phenotypes with loss of motor neurons in spinal cord and brain stem resulting in amyotrophy, fasciculations, weakness that are not linked to SMN gene. They are broadly categorized under the umbrella of spinal muscular atrophy syndromes or hereditary motor neuronopathies or non-5Q-linked spinal muscular atrophy. Several investigators isolated small groups of families with these disorders and linked them to specific chromosome abnormalities. Following are a few to name.

Late Onset Spinal Motor Neuronopathy (LOSMoN)

This is an autosomal-dominant form of SMA first reported by Jokela et al. in two Finnish families (Jokela-type SMA, or SMAJ) [2]. A missense mutation c.197G>T (p.G66V) in the CHCHD10 gene was linked to it. Age of onset was between 25 and 30 years characterized by muscle cramps, fasciculations, and slowly progressive weakness lasting many decades [2].

Scapuloperoneal SMA (SPSMA)

SPSMA is a rare autosomal-dominant neuromuscular disorder characterized by progressive scapuloperoneal atrophy and weakness caused by mutations in the transient receptor potential cation channel subfamily V member 4 gene (TRPV4). The clinical features can range from congenital absence of muscles to progressive scapuloperoneal atrophy, laryngeal palsy, and progressive distal weakness and amyotrophy.

SMA with Lower Extremity Predominance (SMA-LED)

In 2012, Harms et al. identified autosomal-dominant mutations in the DYNC1H1 gene, encoding the dynein heavy chain, in three families with early-onset SMA [3]. The core clinical features included congenital or very early-onset non-progressive weakness, with a typical pattern of predominantly proximal lower-limb involvement. Scoto et al. in 2015 reported on a large series with 30 patients with DYNC1H1 gene mutations. Most of the families in this series had mutations in the tail domain, predominantly located in exon 8, and disease-onset ranged from in utero to late adulthood (one-fifth of patients): 37% presented at birth with lower-limb malformations, including four patients with severe congenital arthrogryposis. Foot deformities and joint contractures were present in half the patients [4–6].

Spinal and Bulbar Muscular Atrophy (X-Linked) (Kennedy's Disease)

This is also a lower motor neuron type disease with early or late adult onset. It is X-linked hereditary motor neuron disease characterized by slowly progressive bulbar and extremity muscle weakness, atrophy, and fasciculation. SBMA is caused by an expanded trinucleotide cytosine–adenine–guanine (CAG) repeat (>38) in the androgen receptor (AR) gene on X chromosome. The disorder rarely affects females, likely due to random X-inactivation. The age of disease onset varies between the second and seventh decade of life and is inversely correlated with the size of the CAG repeat. Its prevalence is estimated to be around 1–2/100,000 population [7–9].

Clinical features are consistent with motor neuron features and androgen insensitivity causing gynecomastia and testicular atrophy. Treatment is supportive [10].

Amyotrophic Lateral Sclerosis (ALS)

ALS is a mixed motor neuron disease, involving both upper and lower motor neurons. It has a male predominance. As of 2011, prevalence of ALS in the United States is 3.9/100,000. Incidence peaks between 60 and 79 years of age [11].

3 Sleep Issues in Motor Neuron Diseases

It is sporadic (85%) in occurrence although a number of lifestyle (smoking, decreased intake of antioxidant containing foods, sedentary lifestyle), environmental (exposure to beta methyl amino L-alanine, "electric" occupations, heavy metals), and heritable factors (C9ORF72 gene, SOD1 gene, TARDBP gene) have been linked [12].

The diagnosis of ALS is largely clinical, supported by electro diagnostic studies in the absence of alternating pathology explaining the clinical history and exam findings. Clinical presentation is variable; muscle weakness most often begins focally in the extremities and spreads to involve contiguous regions. It is very uncommon for ALS patients to have sphincter, sensory or autonomic dysfunction. For unknown reasons, the sacral spinal cord (Onuf's nucleus) is spared in ALS. Minority of ALS patients (1%) present with respiratory failure. ALS can also have concomitant prominent pseudobulbar palsy (pathologic laughter and crying without a correlation to mood), cognitive impairment.

The current two popular criteria for ALS diagnosis include Awaji criteria and revised El Escorial diagnostic criteria.

ALS is broadly classified into sporadic and familial forms. There is also a less popular phenotypic classification based on clinical features, rapidity of progression of symptoms, and age at onset [13].

Phenotypic Variants of ALS

Limb or Spinal Onset
As the name suggests, arm or leg weakness is seen at onset. ALS can sometimes have predominant lower motor neuron involvement or upper motor neuron involvement which supports the concept that progressive muscular atrophy and primary lateral sclerosis, respectively, are a continuum/part of ALS spectrum.

Bulbar Onset
In this type, the initial onset of symptoms can be from bulbar weakness resulting in speech, swallowing problems. Approximately 25% of ALS patients can have bulbar onset [14].

Other symptoms of bulbar onset ALS is sialorrhea.

ALS-Frontotemporal Dementia
This is a variant with cognitive and behavioral dysfunctions predominance resulting from frontotemporal and fronto striatal pathway involvement. Up to 13% of ALS can fall under this phenotype. The presence of executive dysfunction is associated with decreased survival [15].

ALS is a progressive invariably fatal disease with median life expectancy of 2.5–3 years from symptom onset. Time to diagnose ALS from symptom onset averages between 10 and 16 months. The average life expectancy can be lower in ALS patients with bulbar onset, older age, shorter duration of symptoms by the time of diagnosis and reduced forced vital capacity at the time of diagnosis [11].

Riluzole is the only FDA-approved drug used in ALS to prolong survival and ventilator dependence by 2–3 months. Management is symptomatic and involves a multidisciplinary team effort. This includes mood disorders, sleep disorders, physical symptoms management with appropriate pharmacologic agents. Early initiation of noninvasive ventilation in selective patients improves survival.

Monomelic ALS

This is a benign lower motor neuron disease effecting only one limb with a non-progressive course. It is also known as Hirayama disease and predominantly occurs in India, Japan, and other Asian countries [16–19]. It is characterized by unilateral weakness in arm or leg with asymmetric involvement of proximal and distal muscles. The disorder does not spread to other limbs or to other muscles like respiratory and bulbar muscles. Hence, it is benign and carries a good prognosis. This diagnosis is usually considered after ruling out widespread ALS, brachial plexopathy, post-polio syndrome, multifocal neuropathy with conduction block, etc. [19].

Progressive Muscular Atrophy or Sporadic Lower Motor Neuron Syndromes

Progressive muscular atrophy (PMA) is a degenerative lower motor neuron disease in adults. It is sporadic in occurrence. It accounts for 2.5–11% of all motor neuron diseases with a male predominance [20]. Clinically, it is characterized by progressive flaccid weakness, fasciculations, and muscle atrophy with areflexia. It begins as distal muscle weakness in an asymmetric distribution later spreading to other body regions over months to years. Some authors describe PMA as a spectrum of ALS with eventual UMN involvement. Diagnosis requires clinical and electrophysiological features of LMN dysfunction in two or more different myotome regions, evidence of disease progression and the exclusion of other LMN syndromes (LMNS) [18].

Primary Lateral Sclerosis

Primary lateral sclerosis (PLS) is a disorder of progressive upper motor neuron dysfunction. PLS is a rare disorder, representing approximately 1–4% of all patients with motor neuron disease. It is a diagnosis of exclusion ruling out structural, infectious, demyelinating causes of upper motor neuron degeneration presentation [21]. Upper motor neuron type ALS and hereditary spastic paraplegias are the two top differentials. Like PMA, PLS also exists on amyotrophic lateral sclerosis spectrum (mixed upper and lower motor neuron involvement).

It is characterized by the presence of upper motor neuron signs at least 3 years from onset, without any evidence of lower motor neuron dysfunction. Clinical symptoms usually begin in the legs, occasionally they can start in the bulbar region. Clinical signs include spasticity, hyperreflexia, and upper motor neuron pattern weakness. Treatment is symptomatic and can use baclofen (GABA agonist) and tizanidine (alpha 2 agonist) to reduce spasticity.

Summary

Motor neuron disorders are neurodegenerative diseases of upper/and lower motor neurons. They can be childhood or adulthood disorders. They can be familial or sporadic in occurrence. Among childhood motor neuron diseases, SMA is common. It is autosomal recessive, lower motor neuron type disease caused by gene deletion in SMN1. SMA is further divided into different types based on the highest motor milestone that children achieve. Also there is a small subset of SMA phenotypes in whom the involved gene is not SMN1 and they are called SMA syndromes. Over the years, different genes have been isolated in these syndromes. Kennedy's disease (SBMA) is an X-Linked lower motor neuron disease occurring in the early to late adulthood. Owing to its occurrence due to androgen receptor gene mutation, clinically there is gynecomastia and testicular atrophy along with bulbar and limb weakness. ALS is a mixed upper and lower motor neuron disease with different types based on their dominant feature at onset. These include bulbar onset, FTD-ALS type, limb/spinal onset, and monomelic variants. There is also PMA and PLS types which are lower motor neuron and upper motor neuron involvement, respectively, which are thought to be a spectrum on the ALS before they show mixed features. The differentiation is important mainly for prognosis as later ones have better prognosis.

Sleep Issues in Motor Neuron Diseases

Introduction

Motor neuron diseases are neurodegenerative diseases leading to progressive loss of upper or/and lower motor neurons [22]. Various genetic mutations (Super oxide dismutase 1, Sanataxin, Dynactin 1, etc.) are implicated in the loss of neurons secondary to toxic metabolites accumulation [22]. With loss of brain stem and spinal cord neurons, motor neuron disease patients have pharyngeal, laryngeal, diaphragmatic, and accessory respiratory muscle weakness leading to respiratory compromise. Sleep-related hypoventilation syndromes can be the earliest sign of the muscle weakness [23]. Depending on type of motor neuron disease, these muscles are involved at different stages of the disease process. In SMA types 1 and 2, there is early involvement requiring bi-level positive pressure ventilation and mechanical ventilation in severe cases. SMA patients have relative sparing of diaphragm compared to expiratory muscles of ventilation [24].

In ALS, respiratory muscle weakness occurs as the disease progresses; hence, respiratory function predicts survival as well.

Sleep issues in motor neuron diseases can range from sleep fragmentation due to neuropathic pain, muscle cramps, difficulty with attaining a comfortable position (from muscle weakness), pooling of secretions causing frequent awakenings, restless leg syndrome, periodic limb movements to more serious issues related to sleep disordered breathing like hypoventilation, sleep apnea leading to respiratory failure.

The incidence of respiratory abnormalities during sleep increases as motor neuron disease progresses [25].

Pathophysiology of Sleep and Respiratory Issues in Motor Neuron Diseases

Normal respiration begins with rhythmic signal output from respiratory centers located in brain stem (medulla and pons) which project to cervical spinal cord segments supplying diaphragm. The respiratory centers are in turn influenced by peripheral and central chemoreceptors which sense the levels of pH, arterial oxygen, and carbon dioxide. Any disease process that alters this pathway will lead to respiratory difficulties.

Sleep Stages and Alteration with Respiration

During sleep, the upper airway muscle tone is reduced in non-rapid eye movement sleep (NREM) and almost completely abolished in rapid eye movement (REM) sleep. There is also blunting of chemoreceptors which normally respond to reduced O_2 or increased CO_2 by augmenting pharyngeal dilator activity thereby maintaining airway patency [26]. In normal individuals, this physiologic response is compensated by increased diaphragm and increased intercostal muscle activity in order to maintain ventilation. When this compensatory mechanism is compromised due to disorders causing respiratory muscles weakness, hypoxia and hypoventilation will ensue [27].

Upper Airway Resistance

The airway is maintained mainly by tongue, palate, and pharyngeal muscles. Negative pressures generated during inspiration stimulate trigeminal sensory afferents producing a protective increase in pharyngeal muscle tone, preventing upper airway collapse [26].

Bulbar muscle weakness and reduced pharyngeal tone in sleep (particularly in REM sleep) are the key factors for increased upper airway resistance and resultant obstructive sleep apnea (OSA) causing oxygen desaturation. In addition, airway patency can be compromised by other factors including obesity, short neck, tonsillar/adenoid hypertrophy (especially in children), and macroglossia. Combination of increased upper airway resistance, presence of bulbar and/or diaphragm weakness, and associated structural airway abnormalities in patients with motor neuron diseases leads to severe ventilatory deficit during REM sleep [27].

Alterations in Chemo-Sensitivity and Respiratory Control

As mentioned previously, there is physiologic blunting of chemo-receptors during sleep. Chronic hypoventilation results in impaired respiratory chemo-sensitivity and exacerbates ventilatory insufficiency.

Diaphragm Weakness

Unlike daytime, during sleep, ventilation predominantly depends on the diaphragmatic activity. Hence, any disorder causing diaphragm dysfunction either centrally or peripherally causes sleep disordered breathing (SDB)/ventilatory disturbances. They can begin with brief REM-related respiratory disturbances and progress to frank sleep apnea and REM-related hypoventilation. It can progress to involve NREM sleep also and eventually to diurnal respiratory failure.

Sleep Fragmentation
Sleep-related hypoxemia and hypercarbia in patients with motor neuron diseases can cause frequent arousals and sleep fragmentation. Patients with bulbar weakness have weak cough and difficulty with clearing secretions leading to pooling and mucus plugging which can also result in arousals from choking.

Sleep Disorders in Motor Neuron Diseases

Sleep Disordered Breathing (SDB)
Sleep disordered breathing refers to ventilatory disturbances resulting in sleep fragmentation. It is the most common sleep disorder in ALS patients. SDB can be seen in up to three fourths of the ALS patients [28]. SDB can present in a variety of ways including frank sleep apnea, sleep-related hypoventilation, or hypoxia.

Nocturnal Hypoventilation and Hypoxemia
Among SDB, nocturnal hypoventilation is the most prevalent disorder in motor neuron diseases [29].

Nocturnal hypoventilation during sleep is defined as an increase in the arterial $PaCO_2$ to a value greater than or equal to 55 mmHg for greater than or equal to 10 min, or a value greater than or equal to 10 mmHg increase in the arterial $PaCO_2$ relative to the awake supine value, to a value exceeding 50 mmHg for 10 min or more [30].

It occurs when alveolar ventilation is decreased and unable to meet metabolic needs. This is secondary to diaphragm, intercostal and accessory muscle weakness and reduced central drive to respiratory muscles causing inadequate ventilation thereby causing carbon dioxide retention [31].

This can coexist with sleep apnea. The combination of nocturnal hypoventilation and sleep apnea is sometimes called Overlap syndrome [32].

Frequent awakenings and daytime somnolence could be an early sign of respiratory failure from nocturnal hypoventilation in patients with motor neuron disease [28, 33]. With progression of weakness, daytime hypoventilation eventually occurs [34] resulting in orthopnea or exertional dyspnea which may be the presenting symptom in these patients [27].

Sleep Apnea (Obstructive, Central, and Mixed)
Respiratory events in obstructive sleep apnea are characterized by continued thoraco-abdominal effort in the setting of partial or complete airflow cessation, while those in central sleep apnea lack thoraco-abdominal effort [30, 35]. Obstructive sleep apnea syndrome is defined as apnea-hypopnea index of >5/h with associated symptoms (e.g., excessive daytime sleepiness, fatigue, or

impaired cognition) or a AHI of 15 or greater, regardless of associated symptoms [36].

Central apnea and hypoventilation are the most common forms of SDB in ALS patients [6, 29]. Theoretically, it is expected that bulbar form of ALS would have higher incidence of obstructive sleep apnea due to the upper airway muscle weakness. However, previous studies did not demonstrate this pattern [37–40]. OSA has a higher incidence in spinal and bulbar muscular atrophy. Predominant diaphragm or pharyngeal muscle involvement may determine severity of hypoventilation and superimposed central, obstructive, or mixed apneic events.

Restless Leg Syndrome (RLS) and Periodic Leg Movements in Sleep (PLMS)

RLS is defined by the presence of an urge to move the legs, usually accompanied by uncomfortable or unpleasant sensations, which begins or worsens during inactivity, are relieved by movement and usually occur in the evening [41]. RLS is frequently accompanied by the occurrence of periodic leg movements in sleep (PLMS). PLMS occur in approximately 80–90% of patients who have RLS [41]. RLS and PLMS occurrence is higher in ALS patients compared to general population [42, 43]. Daniele Lo coco et al. performed a study in 2010 comparing 76 ALS patients and 100 control subjects and concluded that ALS patients with RLS have a shorter history and higher frequency of symptoms leading to sleep disruption and functional impairment [42]. Same group compared 41 ALS patients and 26 healthy subjects and found 22 patients (53.6%) with a PLMS index >15/h vs. 4 (15.4%) controls. They also noted that 2 patients (4.9%) had RBD, and 2 other patients (4.9%) presented with REM sleep without atonia (RSWA), whereas none of the controls had abnormalities of REM sleep [22].

Insomnia

Insomnia is defined as a subjective report of difficulty with sleep initiation, duration, consolidation, or impaired quality that occurs despite adequate opportunity for sleep, and results in some form of daytime impairment [44]. Insomnia in motor neuron diseases patients is multifactorial. As the disease progresses, the degenerative process leads to muscle atrophy and weakness. This can make even turning in the bed to get into a comfortable position difficult interrupting sleep. Muscle fasciculations, fatigue, cramps, and pain from neuropathy frequently disrupt sleep. With bulbar form, the inability to clear secretions results in pooling and choking during sleep. Mood disturbances secondary to associated depression and anxiety also plays a major part in sleep quality.

Approach to Diagnoses

Comprehensive Sleep History and Clinical Examination

Details about sleep hygiene, sleep initiation, nocturnal arousals, breathing pattern, abnormal movements in sleep, and any personal factors limiting sleep should be inquired in every patient. This should be supplemented by bed partner experiences (Clues for apneic events, PLMS, RBD).

Most commonly reported night time symptoms by motor neuron disease patients are nocturia, sleep fragmentation, and nocturnal cramps.

Daytime complaints pointing towards a sleep disorder in motor neuron disease patients are daytime sleepiness, fatigue, early morning headaches, poor concentration, and memory problems. Any urge to move legs during physical inactivity or in the evenings, discomfort sensation in legs which gets better by moving them can point towards RLS.

A comprehensive history combined with examination findings helps in choosing patients for further diagnostic testing like pulmonary function tests and polysomnogram.

Pulmonary Function Tests

Following motor neuron disease diagnosis, it is important to have baseline pulmonary function testing (PFT) done. PFTs are useful indicators of respiratory involvement, reserve, and disease progression. They guide with initiation of noninvasive ventilation and aid in prognostication as well.

Reduction of FVC (Forced Vital Capacity) and FEV1 (Forced Expiratory Volume in the first second) are predictors of poor survival in ALS patients. PFTs usually show a restrictive pattern in ALS patients. Reductions in supine position FVCs are useful predictors of diaphragm weakness [45].

Nocturnal Pulse Oximetry in Conjunction with Capnography

Night time continuous oxygen monitoring is an easy bed side tool to document nocturnal hypoxemia and could suggest sleep disordered breathing. This is conjunction with a Capnography which measures end tidal carbon dioxide in expired air [46] is an efficient tool for assessing nocturnal hypoventilation. It can also predict good compliance with Noninvasive ventilation treatment for ALS patients [47].

These bed side tools help physicians to screen/prioritize patients for overnight Polysomnogram studies which are gold standard for diagnosing various sleep disorders.

Polysomnogram Study (PSG)

The main indications for PSG in patients with motor neuron diseases are clinical symptoms of SDB, $PaCO_2$ > 45 mmHg on arterial blood gas (ABG), forced vital capacity (FVC) <2.5 kPa [27]. PSG helps with diagnosing sleep disordered breathing and titration of Noninvasive ventilation (NIV) in ALS patients.

Variation in the proportion of obstructive and central apneas/hypopneas, among different studies on patients with similar disease type and severity, may be partly related to the difficulties in classification of the events in the presence of severe weakness. For example, obstructive apneas may be misinterpreted as central events when respiratory muscles are too weak to move the chest wall against the collapsed pharynx. Conversely, severe weakness of the diaphragm may lead to paradoxical movement of the chest and abdomen despite normal upper airway patency, and cause central apneas to be misclassified as obstructive [27].

Sniff Nasal Inspiratory Pressure (SNIP)

A sniff is a short, sharp, voluntary inspiratory maneuver. SNIP is a noninvasive test to assess transdiaphragmatic strength and is sensible to small changes in respiratory function [48]. It consists of measuring nasal pressure through a plug occluding one nostril during a maximal sniff performed through the contralateral nostril [49]. Studies have proven that it correlates well with invasive and nonvolitional diaphragm strength predictor tests [40].

A SNIP <60 cm H_2O could be an early predictor of SDB in ALS patients [50].

The practice parameters update of the American Academy of Neurology added a sniff nasal pressure <40 cm H_2O and orthopnea as additional criteria that may justify initiation of NIV.

Miscellaneous Diagnostics

Phrenic nerve EMG and fluoroscopy can be used to assess diaphragm function [24].

Management

Sleep Hygiene

It involves teaching patients about healthy lifestyle practices that improve sleep. Used in conjunction with stimulus control, relaxation training, sleep restriction, or cognitive therapy, it can also help in management of insomnia.

Instructions include, but are not limited to, keeping a regular sleep-wake schedule, having a healthy diet and regular daytime exercise, having a quiet sleep environment, and avoiding daytime napping, caffeine, other stimulants, nicotine, alcohol, excessive fluids, or stimulating activities before bedtime [44].

Treatment of Comorbid Conditions

Comorbid conditions of hypothyroidism, obesity, congestive heart failure (leading to orthopnea), iron deficiency (that can worsen symptoms of RLS), mood disorders (may cause insomnia), neuropathic pain and cramps leading to sleep fragmentation should all be appropriately addressed.

Pharmacotherapy

Management of Restless Legs Syndrome

Dopamine agonists like ropinirole, pramipexole are standard treatments for RLS. Other treatments include gabapentin, pregabalin, and iron supplements (when ferritin is low). These agents should be used after weighing risks vs. benefits [51].

Management of Insomnia

In insomnia patients, sleep aids, short-intermediate acting benzodiazepine receptor agonists, sedating antidepressants, atypical antipsychotics may be prescribed on a case-by-case basis depending on severity of insomnia, presence or absence of comorbid conditions including mood disorders with insomnia, drug-to-drug interactions [44].

Noninvasive Pressure Ventilation (NIV)

Management of Sleep-Related Breathing Disorder, Hypoventilation, and Hypoxemia

Noninvasive pressure ventilation improves quality and survival in motor neuron disease patients with sleep disordered breathing [24].

Current criteria for Medicare coverage of NIV in patients with ALS include any of: FVC < 50%, maximum inspiratory pressure <60 cm H_2O, SpO_2 ≤ 88% for at least 5 continuous minutes or longer, or a $PaCO_2$ of >45 mm Hg [52].

The practice parameters update of the American Academy of Neurology added a sniff nasal pressure <40 cm H_2O and orthopnea as additional criteria that may justify initiation of NIV.

Boentert et al. demonstrated an increase in SWS, REM sleep, and oxygen saturation (SpO_2) during the early phase of NIV initiation. Mean apnea-hypopnea index, respiratory rate, and the maximum transcutaneous carbon dioxide tension were all reduced [53].

Limitations with NIV

Although NIV is the standard of care for sleep disordered breathing abnormalities, it is sometimes limited by factors such as air leaks, central apneas, glottic closure which lead to desaturations, sleep arousals, and poor compliance. These limitations can be corrected to some extent using PSG for titrating NIV parameters and recognizing sleep disordered breathing events from NIV.

Diaphragm Pacing and Tracheostomy

A preliminary study with diaphragm pacing in 18 ALS patients showed improved sleep efficiency with fewer arousals and micro-arousals [54].

Summary

Motor neuron diseases are a group of neurodegenerative disorders involving gradual loss of upper or lower motor neuron or both in the spinal cord or/and brain stem causing progressive impairment of motor, bulbar, and respiratory function succumbing patients to death from complications related to them.

Good sleep is an essential component of improving quality of life. Diaphragm is the principle contributor for ventilation during sleep. Disorders causing diaphragm weakness such as motor neuron diseases result in sleep hypoventilation syndromes and eventually daytime ventilation difficulties. It is critical for clinicians to recognize subtle signs during sleep which gives a clue about respiratory involvement early on.

A comprehensive history and examination is vital when evaluating and addressing sleep issues in motor neuron diseases. This should be followed by polysomnogram and pulmonary function testing to determine which patients benefit from noninvasive pressure ventilation. Early intervention with noninvasive pressure ventilation has shown to improve survival and quality of life.

Prescription medications for restless leg syndrome, insomnia, sialorrhea, cramps, and mood disturbances should be considered on a case-by-case basis weighing risks vs. benefits.

Key Points
1. Motor neuron diseases are a group of neurodegenerative disorders resulting from upper/and lower motor neurons. They can set in during childhood or in adulthood; while some are rapidly progressive, others can be slowly progressive.
2. SMN in children and ALS in adults is the most prevalent motor neuron disorder in respective age groups.
3. Sleep issues in motor neuron disorders have gained importance over the last few decades as their quality of life can be improved by addressing the issues at appropriate times.
4. Nocturnal hypoventilation, obstructive sleep apnea, and central sleep apnea are the three major contributors of sleep disordered breathing in motor neuron diseases.
5. NIV has shown improved survival and quality of life in ALS patients with sleep disordered breathing.
6. Identifying sleep issues in motor neuron diseases can be challenging and involves a multidisciplinary approach with clinical history, exam, and appropriate diagnostic studies (PSG, PFT, ABG, etc.)
7. Other sleep disorders include RLS, insomnia, mood disorders disrupting sleep, and RBD requiring different pharmacotherapeutic options

References

1. Kolb SJ, Kissel JT. Spinal muscular atrophy. Neurol Clin. 2015;33(4):831–46.
2. Jokela M, Penttila S, Huovinen S, Hackman P, Saukkonen AM, Toivanen J, et al. Late-onset lower motor neuronopathy: a new autosomal dominant disorder. Neurology. 2011;77(4):334–40.
3. Harms MB, Allred P, Gardner R Jr, Fernandes Filho JA, Florence J, Pestronk A, et al. Dominant spinal muscular atrophy with lower extremity predominance: linkage to 14q32. Neurology. 2010;75(6):539–46.
4. Rudnik-Schoneborn S, Deden F, Eggermann K, Eggermann T, Wieczorek D, Sellhaus B, et al. Autosomal dominant spinal muscular atrophy with lower extremity predominance: a recognizable phenotype of BICD2 mutations. Muscle Nerve. 2016;54(3):496–500.
5. Tsurusaki Y, Saitoh S, Tomizawa K, Sudo A, Asahina N, Shiraishi H, et al. A DYNC1H1 mutation causes a dominant spinal muscular atrophy with lower extremity predominance. Neurogenetics. 2012;13(4):327–32.
6. Niu Q, Wang X, Shi M, Jin Q. A novel DYNC1H1 mutation causing spinal muscular atrophy with lower extremity predominance. Neurol Genet. 2015;1(2):e20.
7. La Spada AR, Wilson EM, Lubahn DB, Harding AE, Fischbeck KH. Androgen receptor gene mutations in X-linked spinal and bulbar muscular atrophy. Nature. 1991;352(6330):77–9.
8. Finsterer J. Bulbar and spinal muscular atrophy (Kennedy's disease): a review. Eur J Neurol. 2009;16(5):556–61.

9. Goldenberg JN, Bradley WG. Testosterone therapy and the pathogenesis of Kennedy's disease (X-linked bulbospinal muscular atrophy). J Neurol Sci. 1996;135(2):158–61.
10. Finsterer J, Soraru G. Onset manifestations of spinal and bulbar muscular atrophy (Kennedy's disease). J Mol Neurosci. 2016;58(3):321–9.
11. Statland JM, Barohn RJ, McVey AL, Katz JS, Dimachkie MM. Patterns of weakness, classification of motor neuron disease, and clinical diagnosis of sporadic amyotrophic lateral sclerosis. Neurol Clin. 2015;33(4):735–48.
12. Ingre C, Roos PM, Piehl F, Kamel F, Fang F. Risk factors for amyotrophic lateral sclerosis. Clin Epidemiol. 2015;7:181–93.
13. Al-Chalabi A, Hardiman O, Kiernan MC, Chio A, Rix-Brooks B, van den Berg LH. Amyotrophic lateral sclerosis: moving towards a new classification system. Lancet Neurol. 2016;15(11):1182–94.
14. Chio A, Calvo A, Moglia C, Mazzini L, Mora G, PARALS Study Group. Phenotypic heterogeneity of amyotrophic lateral sclerosis: a population based study. J Neurol Neurosurg Psychiatry. 2011;82(7):740–6.
15. Phukan J, Elamin M, Bede P, Jordan N, Gallagher L, Byrne S, et al. The syndrome of cognitive impairment in amyotrophic lateral sclerosis: a population-based study. J Neurol Neurosurg Psychiatry. 2012;83(1):102–8.
16. Hamano T, Mutoh T, Hirayama M, Kuriyama M. [Benign monomelic amyotrophy]. Ryoikibetsu Shokogun Shirizu. 1999;(27 Pt 2):388–91.
17. Delerue O, Hurtevent JF, Destee A. [Benign, monomelic juvenile amyotrophy of a hand (Hirayama type): a new case report]. Acta Neurol Belg. 1990;90(2):82–6.
18. Drozdowski W, Baniukiewicz E, Lewonowska M. [Juvenile monomelic amyotrophy: Hirayama disease]. Neurol Neurochir Pol. 1998;32(4):943–50.
19. Nalini A, Gourie-Devi M, Thennarasu K, Ramalingaiah AH. Monomelic amyotrophy: clinical profile and natural history of 279 cases seen over 35 years (1976-2010). Amyotroph Lateral Scler Frontotemporal Degener. 2014;15(5-6):457–65.
20. Liewluck T, Saperstein DS. Progressive muscular atrophy. Neurol Clin. 2015;33(4):761–73.
21. Statland JM, Barohn RJ, Dimachkie MM, Floeter MK, Mitsumoto H. Primary lateral sclerosis. Neurol Clin. 2015;33(4):749–60.
22. Dion PA, Daoud H, Rouleau GA. Genetics of motor neuron disorders: new insights into pathogenic mechanisms. Nat Rev Genet. 2009;10(11):769–82.
23. Fermin AM, Afzal U, Culebras A. Sleep in neuromuscular diseases. Sleep Med Clin. 2016;11(1):53–64.
24. Gozal D. Pulmonary manifestations of neuromuscular disease with special reference to Duchenne muscular dystrophy and spinal muscular atrophy. Pediatr Pulmonol. 2000;29(2):141–50.
25. Santos C, Braghiroli A, Mazzini L, Pratesi R, Oliveira LV, Mora G. Sleep-related breathing disorders in amyotrophic lateral sclerosis. Monaldi Arch Chest Dis. 2003;59(2):160–5.
26. Horner RL. Pathophysiology of obstructive sleep apnea. J Cardiopulm Rehabil Prev. 2008;28(5):289–98.
27. Dhand UK, Goyal MK, Sahota PK. Sleep related hypoventilation/hypoxemia due to neuromuscular and chest wall disorders. In: Kushida C, editor. Encyclopedia of sleep. 1st ed: Academic Press; 2012.
28. Gaig C, Iranzo A. Sleep-disordered breathing in neurodegenerative diseases. Curr Neurol Neurosci Rep. 2012;12(2):205–17.
29. Miller RG, Jackson CE, Kasarskis EJ, England JD, Forshew D, Johnston W, et al. Practice parameter update: the care of the patient with amyotrophic lateral sclerosis: drug, nutritional, and respiratory therapies (an evidence-based review): report of the Quality Standards Subcommittee of the American Academy of Neurology. Neurology. 2009;73(15):1218–26.
30. Berry RB, Budhiraja R, Gottlieb DJ, Gozal D, Iber C, Kapur VK, et al. Rules for scoring respiratory events in sleep: update of the 2007 AASM manual for the scoring of sleep and associated events. Deliberations of the Sleep Apnea Definitions Task Force of the American Academy of Sleep Medicine. J Clin Sleep Med. 2012;8(5):597–619.

31. Piper AJ. Nocturnal hypoventilation - identifying & treating syndromes. Indian J Med Res. 2010;131:350–65.
32. Flenley DC. Sleep in chronic obstructive lung disease. Clin Chest Med. 1985;6(4):651–61.
33. Labanowski M, Schmidt-Nowara W, Guilleminault C. Sleep and neuromuscular disease: frequency of sleep-disordered breathing in a neuromuscular disease clinic population. Neurology. 1996;47(5):1173–80.
34. Nicolle MW. Sleep and neuromuscular disease. Semin Neurol. 2009;29(4):429–37.
35. Romigi A, Liguori C, Placidi F, Albanese M, Izzi F, Uasone E, et al. Sleep disorders in spinal and bulbar muscular atrophy (Kennedy's disease): a controlled polysomnographic and self-reported questionnaires study. J Neurol. 2014;261(5):889–93.
36. Sleep-related breathing disorders in adults: recommendations for syndrome definition and measurement techniques in clinical research. The report of an American Academy of Sleep Medicine Task Force. Sleep. 1999;22(5):667–89.
37. Kimura K, Tachibana N, Kimura J, Shibasaki H. Sleep-disordered breathing at an early stage of amyotrophic lateral sclerosis. J Neurol Sci. 1999;164(1):37–43.
38. David WS, Bundlie SR, Mahdavi Z. Polysomnographic studies in amyotrophic lateral sclerosis. J Neurol Sci. 1997;152(Suppl 1):S29–35.
39. Arnulf I, Similowski T, Salachas F, Garma L, Mehiri S, Attali V, et al. Sleep disorders and diaphragmatic function in patients with amyotrophic lateral sclerosis. Am J Respir Crit Care Med. 2000;161(3 Pt 1):849–56.
40. Lyall RA, Donaldson N, Polkey MI, Leigh PN, Moxham J. Respiratory muscle strength and ventilatory failure in amyotrophic lateral sclerosis. Brain. 2001;124(Pt 10):2000–13.
41. Allen RP, Picchietti D, Hening WA, Trenkwalder C, Walters AS, Montplaisi J, et al. Restless legs syndrome: diagnostic criteria, special considerations, and epidemiology. A report from the restless legs syndrome diagnosis and epidemiology workshop at the National Institutes of Health. Sleep Med. 2003;4(2):101–19.
42. Lo Coco D, Piccoli F, La Bella V. Restless legs syndrome in patients with amyotrophic lateral sclerosis. Mov Disord. 2010;25(15):2658–61.
43. Lo Coco D, Puligheddu M, Mattaliano P, Congiu P, Borghero G, Fantini ML, et al. REM sleep behavior disorder and periodic leg movements during sleep in ALS. Acta Neurol Scand. 2017;135(2):219–24.
44. Schutte-Rodin S, Broch L, Buysse D, Dorsey C, Sateia M. Clinical guideline for the evaluation and management of chronic insomnia in adults. J Clin Sleep Med. 2008;4(5):487–504.
45. Javad Mousavi SA, Zamani B, Shahabi Shahmiri S, Rohani M, Shahidi GA, Mostafapour E, et al. Pulmonary function tests in patients with amyotrophic lateral sclerosis and the association between these tests and survival. Iran J Neurol. 2014;13(3):131–7.
46. Bach JR, Bakshiyev R, Hon A. Noninvasive respiratory management for patients with spinal cord injury and neuromuscular disease. Tanaffos. 2012;11(1):7–11.
47. Kim SM, Park KS, Nam H, Ahn SW, Kim S, Sung JJ, et al. Capnography for assessing nocturnal hypoventilation and predicting compliance with subsequent noninvasive ventilation in patients with ALS. PLoS One. 2011;6(3):e17893.
48. Stefanutti D, Benoist MR, Scheinmann P, Chaussain M, Fitting JW. Usefulness of sniff nasal pressure in patients with neuromuscular or skeletal disorders. Am J Respir Crit Care Med. 2000;162(4 Pt 1):1507–11.
49. Miller JM, Moxham J, Green M. The maximal sniff in the assessment of diaphragm function in man. Clin Sci (Lond). 1985;69(1):91–6.
50. Carratu P, Cassano A, Gadaleta F, Tedone M, Dongiovanni S, Fanfulla F, et al. Association between low sniff nasal-inspiratory pressure (SNIP) and sleep disordered breathing in amyotrophic lateral sclerosis: Preliminary results. Amyotroph Lateral Scler. 2011;12(6):458–63.
51. Aurora RN, Kristo DA, Bista SR, Rowley JA, Zak RS, Casey KR, et al. The treatment of restless legs syndrome and periodic limb movement disorder in adults–an update for 2012: practice parameters with an evidence-based systematic review and meta-analyses: an American Academy of Sleep Medicine Clinical Practice Guideline. Sleep. 2012;35(8):1039–62.

52. Clinical indications for noninvasive positive pressure ventilation in chronic respiratory failure due to restrictive lung disease, COPD, and nocturnal hypoventilation–a consensus conference report. Chest. 1999;116(2):521–34.
53. Boentert M, Brenscheidt I, Glatz C, Young P. Effects of non-invasive ventilation on objective sleep and nocturnal respiration in patients with amyotrophic lateral sclerosis. J Neurol. 2015;262(9):2073–82.
54. Gonzalez-Bermejo J, Morelot-Panzini C, Salachas F, Redolfi S, Straus C, Becquemin MH, et al. Diaphragm pacing improves sleep in patients with amyotrophic lateral sclerosis. Amyotroph Lateral Scler. 2012;13(1):44–54.

Sleep Issues in Myopathic Disorders and Muscular Dystrophies

Valentina Joseph, Joe Devasahayam, and Munish Goyal

Introduction

Sleep disorders are frequent in patients with neuromuscular disorders but they are poorly recognized. Even with recognition of these disorders, they are sometimes wrongly attributed to be a consequence of their underlying neuromuscular diseases. With advances in sleep medicine and relatively more patients undergoing polysomnograms (PSG), the knowledge about sleep disorders in this patient population is increasing. Also, early recognition and treatment of sleep disorders have shown to improve not only the quality of life but also the life expectancy in some of these patients.

Common sleep-related complaints are fragmented sleep, breathing difficulty during sleep, abnormal limb movements during sleep, insomnia, muscle pain, early morning headaches, daytime sleepiness, etc. [1].

Common Sleep Disorders in Neuromuscular Disorders

1. Sleep-related breathing disorders
2. Insomnia
3. Sleep-related movement disorders
4. Circadian rhythm sleep-wake disorders
5. Parasomnias

V. Joseph, M.D. (✉)
Neurology and Sleep Medicine, University of South Dakota-Sanford School of Medicine, Sioux Falls, SD, USA

J. Devasahayam, M.D.
University of Missouri, Columbia, MO, USA

M. Goyal, M.D.
Department of Neurology, University of Missouri, Columbia, MO, USA
e-mail: Munishk@health.missouri.edu

Sleep Disordered Breathing in Myopathies and Muscular Dystrophies

Sleep disordered breathing (SDB) are a group of disorders that occur as a result of abnormal breathing pattern during sleep. According to International Classification of Sleep Disorders (ICSD-3), these include obstructive sleep apnea syndromes, central sleep apnea syndromes, sleep-related hypoventilation disorders, and sleep-related hypoxemia disorders. The prevalence of obstructive sleep apnea (OSA) (defined as respiratory disturbance index (RDI) or apnea-hypopnea index (AHI) >5) in healthy adult population was found to be 13% in men and 6% in women [2].

The estimated prevalence of SDB in neuromuscular diseases is about 36–53% in adults [3]. The exact prevalence of SDB in myopathies and muscular dystrophies is not known. However, it is to be noted that this study [3] included patients with Duchenne's muscular dystrophy, myotonic dystrophy along with other congenital and metabolic myopathies. In patients with muscle disease who have SDB, the presence of SDB itself could increase their morbidity and mortality. SDB could be an earlier manifestation in these patients, who eventually may develop respiratory failure [3, 4].

Normal Breathing Pattern During Sleep

Breathing normally varies significantly between wakefulness and sleep, and between supine and upright postures as well. In supine position, there is a mild reduction in inspiratory and expiratory reserve volumes and hence a reduction in the vital capacity and total lung capacity is seen.

During NREM sleep, there is a reduction in respiratory rate, tidal volume, pharyngeal dilator muscle activity, and ventilator drive of wakefulness, resulting in slight increase in the partial pressure of carbon dioxide in blood. In REM sleep, muscle atonia develops. Even though, ventilation is decreased further, due to varied involvement of muscle groups in REM (the pharyngeal and intercostal muscles are affected the most and the diaphragmatic muscles are affected the least), *in a normal individual, the only muscle which is still able to maintain breathing during REM sleep is diaphragm*. Hence, the role of intercostal muscles in NREM and diaphragm in REM are vital [5, 6].

Mechanisms of SDB in Patients with Muscle Disease

Normal functioning of respiratory muscles and diaphragm is essential to carry out breathing during sleep. Their structural integrity and functions are especially important in supine position and in REM sleep. In myopathies and muscular dystrophies, involvement of these muscles and diaphragm makes the patient susceptible for SDB. Reduction in lung volumes and capacities, diaphragmatic weakness, coexisting cardiac abnormalities, and mechanical airway obstruction could be some of the mechanisms that would contribute to the sleep disordered breathing [Fig. 4.1].

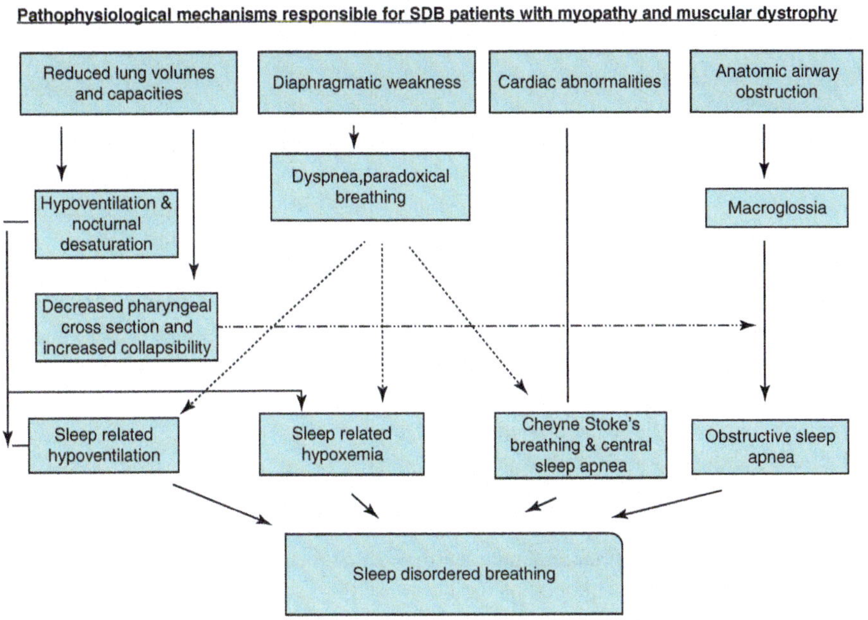

Pathophysiological mechanisms responsible for SDB patients with myopathy and muscular dystrophy

Fig. 4.1 Pathophysiological mechanism responsible for SDB in patients with myopathy and muscular dystrophy

Reduction in Lung Volumes and Capacities

Restrictive ventilatory defect in pulmonary function testing develops once respiratory muscles of the chest wall are involved in the muscle disorders. When compared to normal individuals, these patients have significantly lower inspiratory and expiratory reserve volumes and slightly higher residual volumes. These in turn cause reduction in VC, FRC, and TLC. The lung capacities are much lower in supine position during sleep [6, 7].

The decreased lung capacities are also associated with decrease in pharyngeal airway cross section, due to fall in caudal traction force, further increasing the risk of obstructive sleep apnea [8, 9]. Thus, there are severe nocturnal desaturations especially during REM sleep. The nocturnal pulse oximetry in these patients typically demonstrates a "saw-tooth" pattern. The final result is hypoventilation that leads to chronic hypercarbic respiratory failure [10]. The importance of vital capacity as an independent marker to assess disease progression has already been emphasized in patients with DMD and acid maltase deficiency [4, 15].

Involvement of the Diaphragm

Patients with muscle disease can present with diaphragmatic weakness or paralysis. Clinically, this can cause exertional dyspnea, orthopnea, paradoxical breathing, and recurrent pneumonias [11, 12]. With more understanding of the role of diaphragm in sleep, the sleep pattern in these conditions has been better studied in recent times. These patients tend to have disrupted nocturnal sleep, daytime somnolence, and fatigue. Diaphragmatic weakness has been reported in patients with rigid spine muscular dystrophy [13, 14]. In a study that included 27 subjects with acid maltase deficiency, 13 were found to have diaphragmatic weakness and 12 out of these 13 patients were diagnosed to have SDB in polysomnogram [15]. Diaphragmatic weakness can be a consequence of critical illness myopathy and inflammatory myopathies [16] as well and can pose difficulty in ventilator weaning [17].

Coexisting Cardiac Abnormalities

Cardiac abnormalities are frequently seen in some types of myopathies and muscular dystrophies and contribute significantly towards the mortality in these conditions. Some examples include Emery-Dreifuss muscular dystrophy [18], certain types of Limb-Girdle muscular dystrophy (types 1B, 1D, 2A, 2C, 2E, and 2F), Duchenne's and Becker's muscular dystrophies [19, 20], myotonic dystrophy [21], mitochondriopathies [22], nemaline myopathy [23], and congenital fiber type disproportion [24]. Cardiac manifestations include conduction abnormalities, systolic and diastolic dysfunctions, and intra-cardiac thrombus formation. Cheyne-Stokes breathing can be a consequence of cardiomyopathy in these patients and may be a poor prognostic factor [25].

Anatomical Airway Obstruction

SDB in patients with muscle diseases are usually related to hypoventilation [5]. However, it is also possible to see obstructive sleep pattern in some of these patients. Macroglossia and fibro-fatty replacement of tongue muscles have been reported in patients with acid maltase deficiency (Pompe's disease) leading to obstruction in the airway and OSA [26]. In Duchenne's muscular dystrophy, patients were found to have a bimodal pattern [5] with the increased presence of OSA, at least in the first decade and hypoventilation later on [27–29]. SDB can also occur in both types of myotonic dystrophy with OSA being more common in type 2 (DM2) and central sleep apnea in type 1(DM1) [30, 31].

Insomnia in Myopathies and Muscular Dystrophies

Insomnia is defined as continuing difficulty initiating or maintaining sleep despite enough chances and conditions to sleep, thereby affecting daytime functioning (ICSD-3). In patients with muscle disease, it is not uncommon to see insomnia. The frequent reasons of insomnia in these conditions are muscle pain, hypoventilation/hypercapnia, and also the side effects from medication used to treat these conditions and are listed in Fig. 4.2 below.

Pain is commonly reported in patients with muscle diseases, especially in Duchenne's muscular dystrophy, fascioscapulohumeral muscular dystrophy (FSHD), myotonic dystrophy, and inflammatory myopathies. It is well known that chronic pain/fatigue can cause insomnia and disrupted nocturnal sleep. This has

Fig. 4.2 Causes of insomnia in myopathies and muscular dystrophies

> **Causes of insomnia in myopathies and muscular dystrophies:**
>
> 1) Chronic hypoventilation/ hypercapnia
>
> 2) Muscle pain
>
> 3) Steroid use for treatment of muscle disease

been previously documented in patients with cancer, fibromyalgia, traumatic brain injury, and arthritis [32–36]. Likewise, patients with muscle diseases and muscle pain are also prone to have insomnia. In a case series of four patients with FSHD, all of them were found to have prominent muscle pain in the absence of significant muscle weakness. The muscle pain was severe enough to cause both sleep onset and maintenance insomnia in these patients. In another study which included 55 patients with FSHD, 42 had chronic pain with higher incidence of alpha delta waves during sleep (this alpha intrusion during N3 sleep has been linked with non-restorative sleep) and a reduction in N3 sleep [36, 37].

Insomnia has also been reported in patients with long standing Duchenne's muscular dystrophy who were referred for non-invasive ventilation. Insomnia was thought to be a consequence of chronic hypoventilation and hypercapnia in these patients though other unknown mechanisms are likely to contribute as well [38].

Medicines that are used in the treatment of the muscle conditions can contribute to insomnia. A 6-month prednisone trial in patients with Duchenne's muscular dystrophy, which included 103 patients, showed that these patients had insomnia along with other behavioral symptoms like depression, irritability, and hyperactivity. Sleep-related symptoms were present in 48% of patients who were on prednisone, daily dose of 0.75 mg/kg but increased to 64%, with 1.5 mg/kg dose [39]. This indicates that insomnia could be a dose-dependent side effect of prednisone.

Sleep-Related Movement Disorders

These are disorders in which sleep disturbance is a consequence of simple commonly stereotypical movements that occur either during sleep onset or maintenance. Unlike parasomnias, these disorders do not present with abnormal complex behaviors like eating, walking, dream enactment, etc.

ICSD-3 includes restless legs syndrome (RLS), periodic limb movement disorder (PLMD), sleep-related leg cramps, bruxism, rhythmic movement disorder, and sleep-related movement disorders due to a medical condition, medication/substance use under this category. Of these, RLS is the only disorder that has been reported in patients with muscle diseases specifically in myotonic dystrophy [40].

Restless legs syndrome, also known as Willis-Ekbom disease is a disorder characterized by an uncontrollable need to move the legs, with aggravation of symptoms towards the end of the day and during inactivity. Patients also report complete or limited improvement of symptoms with activity. As a result, the sleep cycle gets disrupted in about 90% of the patients (ICSD-3). In general, RLS can be idiopathic or secondary to some predisposing factors like iron deficiency anemia, pregnancy, chronic renal failure, and medications like antihistamines, dopamine antagonists, and antidepressants except bupropion.

A study done by Mayo clinic which included 30 genetically confirmed myotonic dystrophy type 2 participants(DM2) who were compared with 43 age and sex-matched controls, six patients were found to have RLS symptoms, and three of those had low ferritin levels [40]. Dopamine dysfunction in the striatum and substantia nigra has been linked to the pathophysiology of RLS. Iron being the cofactor for dopamine synthesis, deficiency in iron and ferritin and decreased levels of these in the CSF of these patients is a key factor responsible for causing RLS symptoms [41, 42]. Similarly, in patients with myotonic dystrophy, an RNA toxicity-related abnormal functioning of dopaminergic pathway involving the hypothalamic A11 nuclei is noted [40].

RLS is a clinical diagnosis made if the above-mentioned clinical criteria are met. PSG is not required to diagnose patients with RLS. But, a coexisting finding in PSG which could be noted in patients with RLS is the presence of PLMS and PLMW (periodic limb movements of sleep and wakefulness, respectively). This has been reported in DM2 patients also [40, 42].

RLS has also been reported in a patient with Duchenne's muscular dystrophy who had history of analgesic abuse and chronic pain after taking amitriptyline for chronic pain [43].

Disorders of Central Hypersomnolence

This includes diseases that can present with excessive daytime sleepiness (EDS) and in which the sleepiness is not a consequence of disrupted nocturnal sleep or circadian abnormalities. The disorders included under this category are narcolepsy type 1 and 2, idiopathic hypersomnia, Kleine-Levin syndrome, insufficient sleep syndrome, hypersomnia secondary to medical or psychiatric illness, and hypersomnia secondary to medication or substance use (ICSD-3).

Patients with muscle diseases can have EDS secondary to various reasons like SDB, medication use, etc. But in certain group of patients like myotonic dystrophy, excessive sleepiness can occur in the absence of other factors. The prevalence of EDS could vary between 50% in childhood onset DM and about 70–80% in adult onset patients [44, 45]. A possible "central" etiology wherein structural abnormalities of the cerebral gray and white matter areas have been identified in these patients resulting in daytime sleepiness, cognitive abnormalities, and even depression. Loss of dorsal raphe serotonin producing neurons, which play a vital role in sleep-wake modulation, has also been described in neuropathological analysis. Even though EDS was also noted in DM 2 patients, it was less common than in DM 1. DM 2 patients had higher frequency of depression due to atrophy of limbic region [46].

A narcolepsy-like state with reduced CSF orexin levels was noted in these patients. Unlike narcolepsy with cataplexy, these patients were found to be negative for HLA-DQB1*0602, (a genetic association seen in almost all patients of narcolepsy with cataplexy when compared to general population) and instead patients with DM1 and EDS showed a higher incidence of HLA haplotype DRW6-DQW1 when compared to controls in few studies [47]. In PSG, there was evidence of decreased sleep onset latency and MSLT showed >2 sleep onset REM periods (SOREMPs) which denotes the presence of REM within 15 min of sleep onset (ICSD-3). These findings which are typically seen in patients with narcolepsy were also found in these DM1 patients with narcolepsy-like state. They also showed good treatment response to modafinil [47].

Parasomnias

These are abnormal complex movements associated with behavioral changes, dream enactment, perceptions, and autonomic changes that occur either during sleep onset, maintenance, or during arousal. These disorders can result in physical injuries to the patients or their bed partners. These are classified as NREM and REM parasomnias. NREM parasomnias include confusional arousals, sleepwalking, sleep terrors, and sleep-related eating disorders. REM parasomnias include REM sleep behavior disorder, recurrent isolated sleep paralysis, and nightmare disorder. Figure 4.3 highlights the various different parasomnias.

Even though there are no reports of patients who had history suggestive of any parasomnias, few patients with myotonic dystrophy were found to have increased EMG activity during REM sleep suspicious for REM behavioral disorder. This finding in PSG during REM sleep is called REM sleep without atonia (RSWA) [45, 48].

Circadian Rhythm Disorders

These are disorders that occur due to mismatch between our internal circadian rhythm and outside environment resulting in difficulties with patient's personal and

NREM parasomnias:	REM parasomnias:
- Confusional arousals	- REM sleep behavior disorder
- Sleep walking	- Recurrent isolated sleep paralysis
- Sleep terrors	- Nightmare disorder
- Sleep related eating disorders	

Fig. 4.3 NREM and REM parasomnias

social life. Under this category, some of the disorders included are delayed sleep-wake phase disorder, advanced sleep-wake phase disorder, irregular sleep-wake rhythm disorder, free running disorder or non-24 h sleep-wake rhythm disorder, jet lag disorder, and shift work disorder. To the best of our knowledge, so far there have been no reports of Circadian rhythm disorders in patients with myopathy and muscular dystrophy.

Conclusion

Having understood about the different types of sleep disorders that can occur in patients with muscular dystrophies and myopathies, special attention needs to be given to obtain sleep history in these patients. Appropriate investigations including polysomnograms, MSLT, or even referral to sleep clinics can be considered depending on what type of sleep disorder is suspected.

Key Points
1. Breathing normally varies significantly between wakefulness and sleep, and between supine and upright postures as well.
2. In a normal individual, the only muscle which is still able to maintain breathing during REM sleep is diaphragm.
3. When compared to normal individuals, patients with muscle disease have significantly lower inspiratory and expiratory reserve volumes and slightly higher residual volumes. These in turn cause reduction in VC, FRC, and TLC.
4. The decreased lung capacities are also associated with decrease in pharyngeal airway cross section, due to fall in caudal traction force, further increasing the risk of obstructive sleep apnea.
5. The frequent reasons of insomnia in patients with muscular dystrophy and myopathy are muscle pain, hypoventilation/hypercapnia, and also the side effects from steroid use.
6. A narcolepsy-like state with reduced CSF orexin levels was noted in myotonic dystrophy patients.
7. Few patients with myotonic dystrophy were found to have increased EMG activity during REM sleep suspicious for REM behavioral disorder. This finding in PSG during REM sleep is called REM sleep without atonia (RSWA).
8. In patients with myotonic dystrophy, an RNA toxicity-related abnormal functioning of dopaminergic pathway involving the hypothalamic A11 nuclei is noted, which might contribute to RLS symptoms.
9. A possible "central" etiology wherein structural abnormalities of the cerebral gray and white matter areas have been identified in myotonic dystrophy patients resulting in daytime sleepiness, cognitive abnormalities, and even depression.
10. Appropriate investigations including polysomnogram MSLT or even referral to sleep clinics can be considered depending on what type of sleep disorder is suspected.

References

1. Fermin AM, Afzal U, Culebras A. Sleep in neuromuscular diseases. Sleep Med Clin. 2016;11(1):53–64. https://doi.org/10.1016/j.jsmc.2015.10.005.Epub2016Jan9.
2. Peppard PE, Young T, Hla KM. Increased prevalence of sleep-disorderd breathing in adults. Am J Epidemiol. 2013;177(9):1006–14.
3. Arens R, Muzumdar H. Sleep, Sleep disordered breathing, and nocturnal hypoventilation in children with Neuromuscular diseases. Pediatr Respir Rev. 2010;11(1):24.
4. Phillips MF, Smith PE, Carroll N, Calverley PM. Nocturnal oxygenation and prognosis in Duchenne muscular dystrophy. Am J Respir Crit Care Med. 1999;160(1):198–202.
5. Aboussouan LS. Sleep-disordered breathing in neuromuscular disease. Am J Respir Crit Care Med. 2015;191(9):979–89.
6. Hudgel DW, Devadatta P. Decrease in functional residual capacity during sleep in normal humans. J Appl Physiol. 1984;57:1319–22.
7. Ibanez J, Raurich JM. Normal values of functional residual capacity in the sitting and supine positions. Intensive Care Med. 1982;8:173–7.
8. Appleberg J, Nordahl G, Janson C. Lung volume and its correlation to nocturnal apnoea and desaturation. Respir Med. 2000;94:233–9.
9. Van de Graff WB. Thoracic influence on upper airway patency. J Appl Physiol (1985). 1988;65:2124–31.
10. White JE, Drinnan MJ, Smithson AJ, Griffiths CJ, Gibson GJ. Respiratory muscle activity and oxygenation during sleep in patients with muscular weakness. Eur Respir J. 1989;2:26–30.
11. Smith PE, Edwards RH, Claverly PM. Mechanisms of sleep-disordered breathing in chronic neuromuscular disease: implications for management. Q J Med. 1991;81:961–73.
12. McCool FD, Tzelepis GE. Dysfunction of the diaphragm. N Engl J Med. 2012;366:932–42.
13. Shahrizaila N, Kinnear WJM, Wills AJ. Respiratory involvement in inherited primary muscle conditions. J Neurol Neurosurg Psychiatry. 2006;77(10):1108–15.
14. Ferrerio A, Quijano-Roy S, Piche C. Mutations of the Selenoprotein N gene, which is implicated in rigid spine muscular dystrophy, cause the classical phenotype of multiminicore disease: reassessing the nosology of early-onset myopathies. Am J Hum Genet. 2002;71(4):739–49. https://doi.org/10.1086/342719.
15. Mellies U, Ragette R, Schwake C. Sleep disordered breathing and respiratory failure in acid maltase deficiency. Neurology. 2001;57(7):1290–5.
16. Teixeira A, Cherin P, Similowski T. Diaphragmatic dysfunction in patients with idiopathic inflammatory myopathies. Neuromuscul Disord. 2005;15(1):32–9. https://doi.org/10.1016/j.nmd.2004.09.006.
17. Latronico N, Bolton C. Critical illness polyneuropathy and myopathy: a major cause of muscle weakness and paralysis. Lancet Neurol. 2011;10(10):931–41. https://doi.org/10.1016/S1474-4422(11)70178-8.
18. Madej-Pilarczyk A, Kochanski A. Emery-Dreifuss muscular dystrophy: the most recognizable laminopathy. Folia Neuopathol. 2016;54(1):1–8.
19. Sveen M-L, Thune JJ, Keber L. Cardiac involvement in patients with Limb-Girdle Muscular Dystrophy Type 2 and Becker muscular dystrophy. Arch Neurol. 2008;65(9):1196–201. https://doi.org/10.1001/arch-neur.65.9.1196.
20. van der Kooi AJ, Van Meegen M, Bolhuis PA. Genetic localization of a newly recognized autosomal dominant limb-girdle muscular dystrophy with cardiac involvement (LGMD1B) to chromosome 1q11-21. Am J Hum Genet. 1997;60:891–5.
21. Perloff JK, Stevenson WG, Weiss J. Cardiac involvement in myotonic muscular dystrophy: a prospective study of 25 patients. Am J Cardiol. 1984;54(8):1074–81. https://doi.org/10.1016/S0002-9149(84)80147-2.
22. Zhang LH, Fang LG, Cheng ZW, Fang Q. Cardiac manifestations of patients with mitochondrial disease. Zhonghua Xin Xue Guan Bing Za Zhi. 2009;37(10):892–5.

23. Muller-Hocker J, Schafer S, Mendel B, Lochmuller H, Pongratz D. Nemaline cardiomyopathy in a young adult: an ultraimmunohistochemical study and review of literature. Ultrastruct Pathol. 2000;24(6):407–16.
24. Banwell BL, Becker LE, Jay V, et al. Cardiac manifestations of congenital fiber-type disproportion myopathy. J Child Neurol. 1999;14(2):83–7.
25. Lanfranchi PA, Braghiroli A, Giannuzzi P. Prognostic value of nocturnal Cheyne-Stokes respiration in chronic heart failure. Circulation. 1999;99:1435–40.
26. Muller C, Jones H, O'Grady G, Suzrez A, Heller J, Kishnani P. Language and speech function in children with infantile Pompe disease. J Pediatr Neurol. 2009;7:147–56.
27. Renard D, Humbertclaude V, Labauge P. Macroglossia in adult Duchenne muscular dystrophy. Acta Neurol Belg. 2010;110:288.
28. Khan Y, Heckmatt JZ. Obstructive apnoeas in Duchenne muscular dystrophy. Thorax. 1994;49:157–61.
29. Suresh S, Wales P, Cooper DG. Sleep-related breathing disorder in Duchenne muscular dystrophy: disease spectrum in pediatricpopulation. J Paediatr Child Health. 2005;41:500–3.
30. Leonardis L, Blague R, Dolenc Groselj L. Sleep and breathing disorders in myotonic dystrophy type 2. Acta Neurol Scand. 2015;132:42–8.
31. Bianchi MLE, Losurdo A, Silvestri G. Prevalence and clinical correlates of sleep disordered breathing in myotonic dystrophy types 1 and 2. Sleep Breath. 2014;18:579–89. https://doi.org/10.1007/s11325-013-0921-5.
32. Beetar JT, Guilmette TJ, Sparadeo FR. Sleep and pain complaints in symptomatic traumatic brain injury and neurologic populations. Arch Phys Med Rehabil. 1996;77(12):1298–302.
33. Hoffman AJ, Given BA, Von Eye A. Relationships among pain, fatigue, insomnia and gender in persons with lung cancer. Oncol Nurs Forum. 2007;34(4):785–92.
34. Jennum P, Drewes AM, Andreasen A, Nielsen KD. Sleep and other symptoms in primary fibromyalgia and in healthy controls. J Rheumatol. 1993;20(10):1756–9.
35. Power JD, Perrucio AV, Badley EM. Pain as a mediator of sleep problems in arthritis and other chronic conditions. Arthritis Rheum. 2005;53(6):911–9.
36. Della Marca G, Frusciante R, Vollono C, Ricci E. Pain and the alpha-sleep anomaly: a mechanism of sleep disruption in fascioscapulohumeral muscular dystrophy. Pain Med. 2013;14(4):487–97. https://doi.org/10.1111/pme.12054.
37. Bushby KM, Pollitt C, Johnson MA, Chinnery PF. Muscle pain as a prominent feature of FSHD: four illustrative case reports. Neuromuscul Disord. 1998;8(8):574–9.
38. Vianello A, Bevilacqua M, Vincenti E. Long-term nasal intermittent positive pressure ventilation in advanced Duchenne's muscular dystrophy. Chest. 1994;105(2):445–8.
39. Mendell JR, Moxley RT, Florence J. Randomized, double-blind six-month trial of prednisone in Duchenne's muscular dystrophy. N Engl J Med. 1989;320(24):1592–7.
40. Lam EM, Shepard PW, Milone M. Restless legs syndrome and daytime sleepiness are prominent in myotonic dystrophy type 2. Neurology. 2013;81(2):157–64. https://doi.org/10.1212/WNL.0b013e31829a340f.
41. Ekbom K, Ulfberg J. Restless legs syndrome. J Intern Med. 2009;266(5):419–31. https://doi.org/10.1111/j.1365-2796.2009.02159.
42. Salas RE, Gamaldo CE, Allen RP. Update in restless legs syndrome. Curr Opin Neurol. 2010;23(4):401–6. https://doi.org/10.1097/WCO.0b013e32833bcdd8.
43. Akamine RT, Grossklauss LF, Tufik S. Restless leg syndrome exacerbated by amytriptiline in a patient with Duchenne muscular dystrophy. Sleep Sci. 2014;7(3):178–80. https://doi.org/10.1016/j.slsci.2014.09.010. Epub 2014 Sep 27
44. Dauvilliers YA, Laberge L. Myotonic dystrophy type 1, daytime sleepiness and REM sleep dysregulation. Sleep Med Rev. 2012;16(6):539–45. https://doi.org/10.1016/j.smrv.2012.01.001. Epub 2012 Mar 31
45. Yu H, Laberge L, Dauvilliers Y. Daytime sleepiness and REM sleep characteristics in myotonic dystrophy: a case-control study. Sleep. 2011;34(2):165–70.

46. Schneider-Gold C, Bellenberg B, Lukas C. Cortical and subcortical grey and white matter atrophy in myotonic dystrophies type 1 and 2 is associated with cognitive impairment, depression and daytime sleepiness. PLoS One. 2015;10(6):e0130352.
47. Romigi A, Albanese M, Massa R. Sleep-wake cycle and daytime sleepiness in the myotonic dystrophies. J Neurodegener Dis. 2013;2013:692026.
48. Chokroverty S, Bhat S, Rosen D, Farheen A. REM behavior disorder in myotonic dystrophy type 2. Neurology. 2012;78(24):2004. https://doi.org/10.1212/WNL.0b013e318259e28c.

5

Sleep Issues in Neuromuscular Junction Disorders

Prashant Natteru, Siva Pesala, Pradeep C. Bollu, and Raghav Govindarajan

The Neuromuscular Junction

The neuromuscular junction (NMJ) is a nerve-muscle synapse between a motor neuron and a skeletal muscle fiber. It is a part of the peripheral motor system, which includes the motor neuron within the anterior horn of the spinal cord, the peripheral nerve, the neuromuscular junction, and the muscle distal to it. It forms an essential component of electrical signaling from the nerve cell to the muscle cell. The chemical signaling at these synapses involves the activation of the presynaptic membrane, release of neurotransmitters resulting in opening of ion channels in the postsynaptic membranes [1, 2].

The myelin sheath on the motor neuronal axon terminates near the surface of the muscle fiber, where the unmyelinated axon divides into a number of fine branches. These fine branches form *synaptic boutons*—the point of neurotransmitter release from the presynaptic motor neuron. Each of these presynaptic boutons contains synaptic vesicles of acetylcholine (ACh), and the *active zone*. These active zones are positioned over *junctional folds*—the sockets on the surface of the postsynaptic muscle fiber holding the acetylcholine transmitter receptors (AChR). This region of the muscle cell membrane or the sarcolemma, where the axon terminates to innervate the muscle is called the *end-plate* [1–3]. Figure 5.1 shows the motor end-plate and the neuromuscular junction.

P. Natteru, M.D.
Department of Neurology, University of Mississippi Medical Center, Jackson, MS, USA
e-mail: pnatteru@umc.edu

S. Pesala, M.D. (✉) · P. C. Bollu, M.D. · R. Govindarajan, M.D., F.A.A.N., F.I.S.Qua
Department of Neurology, University of Missouri, Columbia, MO, USA
e-mail: pesalas@health.missouri.edu; BolluP@health.missouri.edu; govindarajanr@health.missouri.edu

© Springer International Publishing AG, part of Springer Nature 2018
R. Govindarajan, P. C. Bollu (eds.), *Sleep Issues in Neuromuscular Disorders*,
https://doi.org/10.1007/978-3-319-73068-4_5

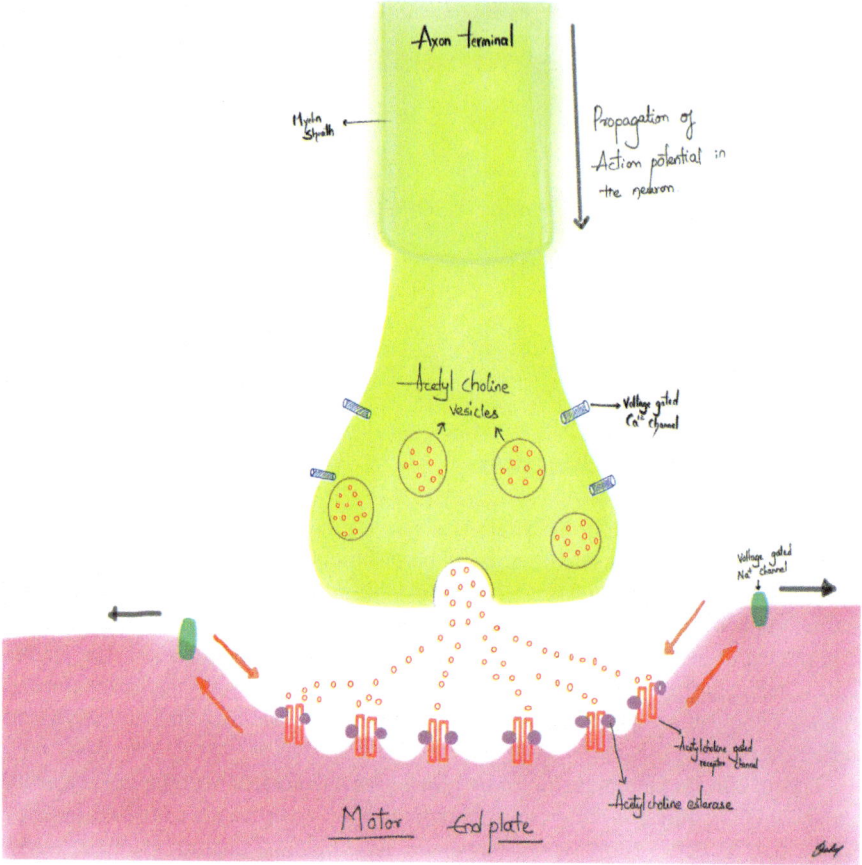

Fig. 5.1 Neuromuscular junction

The end-plate membrane undergoes depolarization, upon the release of acetylcholine from the synaptic clefts. This depolarization produces a large amplitude *end-plate potential* (EPP) in the muscle cell, which activates the voltage-gated Na$^+$ channels in the junctional folds. This synaptic potential at the end-plate rises rapidly, but decays slowly. The sudden release of ACh into the synaptic cleft is the reason for the initial rapid rise. After the release, some of the ACh is quickly removed from the synaptic cleft by acetylcholinesterase (AChE)—a hydrolytic enzyme in the collagen fibrils of the *active zone*, and the remaining diffuses out of the synaptic cleft. Figure 5.1 shows the motor end-plate along with the acetylcholine receptors on it.

The typical end-plate potential is about −30 mV and lasts for 5–10 ms. It brings the adjacent non-end-plate region of the membrane to and above the threshold, which propagates the action potential throughout the length of the muscle fiber. Normally, one nerve action potential → one end-plate potential → one muscle fiber action potential → a single twitch. All of the muscle fibers in a given motor unit are of the same fiber type (all-slow or fast).

Clinical Correlates

(a) Organophosphates inhibit the enzyme acetylcholinesterase → prolong acetylcholine lifetime and its accumulation.
(b) Physostigmine and neostigmine are reversible inhibitors of acetylcholinesterase.
(c) Succinylcholine is a depolarizing muscle relaxant that mimics acetylcholine. It is not readily broken down by acetylcholinesterase, thus causing the initial opening and then inactivation through desensitization of the channel.
(d) Local anesthetics like procaine inhibit the voltage-gated Na^+ channels interfering with the action potential transmission of the nerve.
(e) Botulinum toxin blocks the release of acetylcholine from the nerve terminals.
(f) Hemicholinium decreases acetylcholine production and storage by inhibiting the uptake of choline into the nerve [1–3].

Disorders of the Neuromuscular Junction

Now that the physiology of the neuromuscular junction has been well understood, let us now focus on the disorders of the neuromuscular junction. NMJ disorders are generally pure motor syndromes, which are preferential to the extraocular, proximal, or bulbar muscles. Most of the NMJ disorders are uncommon, but certain conditions like Myasthenia Gravis (MG), Lambert–Eaton myasthenic syndrome (LEMS), and botulism are commonly encountered.

In this section, we will discuss myasthenia gravis and Lambert–Eaton myasthenic syndrome in detail, while also briefly touching upon botulism.

Myasthenia Gravis

The name "Myasthenia" has a Greek origin, whereas "gravis" is Latin, which is literal for *grave muscle weakness*. It is a chronic antibody mediated autoimmune neuromuscular disease, due to an autoantibody against the postsynaptic nicotinic acetylcholine receptor (AChR) or muscle-specific tyrosine kinase (MuSK) at the neuromuscular junction of skeletal muscles. It is characterized by varying weakness of the skeletal (voluntary) muscles of the body [4].

Epidemiology
The clinical axiom of MG being a "disease of young women and old men" stems from the fact that the median age of onset was 41.7 years in women and 60.3 years

for men. A bimodal age distribution was observed in both genders, with the initial peak between 20 and 29 years, and a later steady rise above 50 years. The initial peak was just more pronounced in women [5, 6].

The average age along with the number of late-onset myasthenia gravis patients tends to be on the rise. The number of early-onset myasthenia gravis patients seems unchanged over the years. Within the late-onset MG patients, men and women are affected equally; however, in early-onset MG, women are affected three times more than men. Also, the disease severity, complications, and side effects of treatment are greater in the late-onset group. MuSK myasthenia, on the other hand, was more common in women [7].

Myasthenia gravis patients are associated with a greater incidence of various autoimmune disorders, like thyroid disease, rheumatoid arthritis, and SLE, especially common in first-degree relatives. Other autoimmune diseases commonly associated are pernicious anemia and pemphigus [8].

What Causes Myasthenia Gravis?

Most (80–85%) of the patients with myasthenia gravis have antibodies against the acetylcholine receptor (AChR) in the serum and IgG at the junction. However, about 10% of the myasthenia gravis patients do not demonstrate antibodies against AChR in the serum, and are termed as "seronegative MG."

The AChR antibodies are majorly *binding*, followed by *blocking* (10%) and *modulating* (1%) type.

On an average, about 10% of all patients with myasthenia gravis will have antibodies against muscle-specific tyrosine kinase (MuSK). MuSK is a muscle membrane protein involved in acetylcholine receptor clustering. The characteristic feature of anti-MuSK MG is the significant atrophy of the muscles. Lipoprotein-related protein 4 (LRP4), an agrin receptor involved in agrin activated MuSK and AChR clustering, plays an essential role in the neuromuscular junction formation. Antibodies against LRP4 have been noticed in seronegative MG patients, whereas antibodies against agrin were seen in both seronegative MG and MG patients with anti-AChR.

Thymus gland in MG is almost always abnormal; 85% of the times with thymic hyperplasia (multiple lymphoid follicles with germinal centers), and in about 15% a benign encapsulated thymoma.

Thymomas usually occur in older patients, but can be seen in ages 20–29 years in about 15% of the population.

Clinical Features

Myasthenia gravis can present at any age after birth, with the acquired form being more common. Acquired MG has to be differentiated from transient neonatal myasthenia, which occurs in 10–15% of congenital myasthenia and in children of myasthenic mothers. Transient neonatal myasthenia becomes apparent in the first few years of life.

The Course
The weakness varies from day to day, and sometimes within minutes. Major variations in the course are coined as remissions or exacerbations, and when exacerbations cause respiratory compromise to a degree of needing intubation and mechanical ventilation, it is a myasthenic crisis. This crisis is life threatening, and necessitates aggressive treatment [9]. Children with myasthenia gravis can be tipped into a crisis, due to various respiratory infections. There are certain exacerbating factors like thyroid disease, infectious diseases with fever, psychological stress, certain drugs like antimalarials (quinine, chloroquine), aminoglycosides, D-penicillamine, and beta-blockers [10].

Pregnancy can either improve, worsen, or have no influence on the course of myasthenia gravis [11]. Higher temperatures have been reported to worsen MG, but some of the patients do considerably well in warm weather [12].

The Symptoms
The most frequent manifestations of myasthenia gravis are the ocular symptoms. The ocular muscles are affected early in about 40% of the patients. The involvement of the levator palpebrae superioris along with the extraocular muscles in isolation or in total is the causative factor for vertical, horizontal, diagonal double vision, complete ophthalmoplegia in one or both eyes, or a pattern resembling internuclear ophthalmoplegia (INO). The usual complaint in the majority is of both ptosis and diplopia. Other common symptoms are dysarthria, limited facial movements, and dysphagia due to involvement of oropharyngeal or facial muscles. The characteristic expressionless facial appearance with drooping eyelids is due to the weakness of the levator palpebrae along with the facial muscles [13].

An easy bedside test for the muscles of articulation is by asking the patient to read out loud. Sometimes, dysarthria is accompanied by difficulties in chewing and swallowing, along with regurgitation of liquids through the nose, which is a sign of palatal weakness. Patients who complain of dysphagia describe the sensation of food sticking in the throat, and have a preference for cold food. A possible explanation for this preference is that there may be an improvement in the neuromuscular transmission by cooling of the muscles relatively. Severity of the dysphagia can sometimes correlate with the amount of weight loss. Orbicularis oris weakness results in the inability to kiss, whistle, or in slurping the soup. Some patients complain of excessive meal times, as the time needed for eating a meal increases.

Weakness of the tongue can be tested by asking the patient to push against the inner cheek, or by protruding it out to reach the frenulum of the upper lip. Masticatory muscles can be tested by asking the patient to open and close their mouths repeatedly, until an audible click is heard. Normally, this can be easily performed about a hundred times in 30 s. Weakness of the neck flexors and extensors result in a head drop.

In about 15–20% of the patients, weakness of arms, hands, or legs were the early complaints. Weakness of the legs causes frequent falls and difficulty in climbing stairs, whereas weakness of the upper limbs usually presents with difficulty in going about the daily chores like hanging laundry, or combing hair due to the inability to maintain the arm position above the head.

MuSK myasthenia particularly involves ocular, facial, and bulbar muscles, and carries a high risk of respiratory insufficiency. MuSK myasthenia can follow a rapidly progressive and more severe course.

Most patients complain of excessive fatigability and a feeling of heaviness if the trunk muscles are involved. Due to insufficiency of the postural muscles, sometimes patients experience pain in the back and girdle muscles, which usually resolves with rest.

Respiratory muscle involvement as the very first sign is rare, but respiratory compromise may be the presenting feature to the emergency room in children with a coexisting infection. MuSK myasthenia in particular involves the facial, ocular, and bulbar muscles. It follows a rapidly progressive and severe course due to high risk of respiratory insufficiency.

If a patient is suspected of MG, then the emphasis has to be on testing the muscle strength after exercise for weakness, and not fatigue!

Simple maneuvers are used to test the muscle strength and exhaustibility.

(a) For the arms, hands, and fingers strength: Stretch the arms horizontally, and maintain at the same position for 3 min. Test the strength both pre- and post-stretching. Increasing weakness will produce some drooping of the arms, hands, or fingers. Other neuromuscular disorders will also cause drooping, but the strength pre- and post-stretching would be the same.
(b) Rising from a standard chair repeatedly for about 20 times without using the arms, walking on tiptoes or on heels for at least 30 steps, and straight leg raising to 45° for a minute can aid in assessing the strength in the lower limbs.
(c) Respiratory assessment should include vital capacity, inspiratory and expiratory pressures. Routine pulmonary function tests in MG have shown that the reduction in the vital capacity is far greater than the forced expiratory volume [14].

Localized muscle atrophy is rare, but has been reported in about 6–10% of the patients, especially atrophy of the tongue, shoulder, forearm muscles, and the foot extensors. Sensation and the reflexes are preserved, even in patients with atrophy.

Myasthenic crisis (MC) can be provoked by various factors like a surgical procedure, or a respiratory infection, and sometimes can occur without any provocation. It is a complication of MG causing respiratory compromise and failure, and would need intubation and assisted ventilation. In postsurgical patients, myasthenic crisis can be a reason for prolonged extubation due to flaring up of the muscle weakness in patients with MG. MC normally is expected to occur within the first 2 years after myasthenia gravis onset [13].

Diagnosis

(a) Clinical: The picture of fluctuating weakness improved with rest is a tell-tale sign towards the diagnosis of myasthenia gravis. The bedside ice test can be performed in patients with symptoms suggestive of ocular MG. Resolution of ptosis after the application of a pack of ice over the ptotic eye for 1–2 min is highly specific for MG.

The other test is called TENSILON test, where a short acting acetylcholinesterase (AChE) inhibitor edrophonium will cause an improvement in the muscle weakness of MG within 30–45 s, and sometimes the response lasts up to 5 min. This test should be done under close monitoring with atropine at the bedside, because of the risk of ventricular fibrillation and bradyarrhythmias. Sensitivity is about 60%, and this test can be falsely positive in motor neuron diseases [8].

(b) Laboratory and Electrodiagnostic testing: Antibodies to AChR are seen in 85–90% of patients with generalized MG, and it is the binding type which is most common. In ocular MG, antibodies might not be detected in 50% of the patients. The antibody titer is not a correlate for the disease severity. In a majority (85%) of the patients with thymoma, antibodies to myofibrillar proteins (actin, myosin, actomyosin, titin) are seen. Fifty percent of the seronegative MG has antibodies to MuSK. Like previously mentioned, anti-MuSK MG have predominantly bulbar, facial weakness, with poor response to immunosuppressants, pyridostigmine, thymectomy; and promising response to plasmapheresis. Blood, urine, and CSF workup are usually normal.

Electrodiagnostic testing is important in the diagnosis of MG. Progressive reduction in the amplitude of compound muscle action potentials (CMAPs) by a slow (3–5 Hz) repetitive nerve stimulation (RNS) is typical of MG. This decrement in response to the RNS is the electrical correlate of muscle weakness and fatigability clinically, and can be demonstrated in 90% of the patients using the ulnar-hypothenar, median-thenar, and accessory-trapezius systems. RNS is often abnormal in 50–70% of the patients with generalized MG and can be normal in patients with localized ocular MG.

Treatment

There are numerous treatment options for myasthenia gravis, and based on the individual patient profile, the treatment can be tailored. Let us dwell into the various treatment options available for MG.

(a) Acetylcholinesterase inhibitor (AChEI): These inhibit the hydrolysis of acetylcholine, thereby prolonging the availability of ACh at the NMJ. The most commonly used agent is pyridostigmine bromide. Other agents like neostigmine bromide, neostigmine methylsulfate, and mytelase chloride can be used. Pyridostigmine can be started at 30–60 mg, with dosing intervals between 3 and 6 h. Over time, the beneficial effect of AChE inhibition starts wearing off, and that's when the AChE inhibitors need to be tapered off.

In general, treatment with an AChEI is considered safe, but sometimes, side effects can occur. The usual side effects encountered are nausea, vomiting, diarrhea, abdominal cramps, muscle twitches, cramps, and fasciculations. Atropine and glycopyrrolate can alleviate the GI symptoms, whereas stretching exercises and reassurance can help with the abnormal movements. Bradycardia and confusion can result from AChEI therapy though it is extremely rare. One of the things to watch out for is *cholinergic crisis*, and in patients suspected of having it, discontinuation of AChEI therapy is recommended.

(b) Corticosteroids: They are the most reliable, faster acting of the maintenance therapies available. They are used in patients with generalized weakness, not improved by AChEI; and also patients with bulbar or respiratory weakness. There are various ways in which corticosteroids play a therapeutic role in MG. They alter the lymphokine function, along with reducing their differentiation and proliferation. They also inhibit the function of macrophages, antigen processing and presentation in particular.

When corticosteroids are started on patients, the weakness can worsen during the initial week, followed by improvement, usually by 2 weeks but can take 2–6 months too. To counter the initial worsening of the weakness, plasma exchange can be coupled with steroid therapy. Corticosteroids are administered as a single morning dose to mimic the morning peak of cortisol, and an alternate day regimen is the preferred approach. The side effect profile of corticosteroid therapy includes osteoporosis, glaucoma, cataracts, central obesity, peripheral edema, sleep disturbances, easy bruising, glucose intolerance, depression, mania, and personality alterations.

Vitamin D supplements, calcium, and bisphosphonates are used to counter osteoporosis. For cataracts and glaucoma, yearly ophthalmological evaluation is mandated. Gastric ulcer prophylaxis can be started in patients with gastric irritation. Serum potassium and glucose along with blood pressure needs to be closely monitored. AChR antibody levels trend down within the first few months of initiation of steroid therapy.

(c) Azathioprine: It is a purine analog that inhibits the synthesis of nucleic acids. The cytotoxic metabolite of azathioprine is 6-thioguanine, and it has an immunosuppressive effect on T- and B-cell proliferation. It can be used alone or in combination with corticosteroids. It is often utilized for its corticosteroid-sparing effect, usually noticed after more than a year of treatment. The dose is initiated based on body weight (1–3 mg/kg/day). About 10% of the patients develop fever and flu like symptoms within the first 2 weeks of initiating the treatment. Always be on the lookout for the level of the white blood count, and it has to be maintained above 3500 cells/mm^3. The other parameter worth a mention is the transaminase levels. Azathioprine should be discontinued if transaminases level double [15, 16].

(d) Cyclosporine A: In patients with severe MG who are poor responders to corticosteroids and thymectomy, cyclosporine in doses of 5 mg/kg/day in two doses is recommended. While on cyclosporine, creatinine should be monitored as there is a risk of renal insufficiency, more in elderly. It acts exclusively on T cells and interrupts with the synthesis of cytokines (IL-2 and its surface receptors) [17, 18].

(e) Mycophenolate mofetil (MM): Usually used in the treatment of transplant rejection. Acts on the proliferation of T and B cells by interrupting guanosine synthesis through the inhibition of inosine monophosphate. The other mechanisms include apoptosis of T-lymphocytes, reduced recruitment of lymphocytes, and nitric oxide synthase inhibition.

It is administered at a standard dose of 1 g twice daily. Known adverse effects are GI upset, anemia, and leukopenia. Some studies have shown that MM can be associated with lymphoma, and teratogenicity [19–21].

(f) Tacrolimus (FK 506): It is a macrolide that modulates T-cells by accelerating the apoptotic process. It can replace cyclosporine and decrease the medication-related complications. FK 506 is known to be hepatotoxic, nephrotoxic, and can cause paresthesias. In patients with hypertension and diabetes, it may worsen their condition [22].

(g) Plasma Exchange (Plasmapheresis): Regardless of seropositivity, plasma exchange brings about an instantaneous improvement in myasthenic weakness. Majorly used in myasthenic crisis. Regularly, about 5–6 exchanges are needed. It causes an immediate improvement within 48 h of initiating the exchange, and the levels of the antibodies against AChR drop rapidly. Sometimes, this drop can be followed by a rebound in a few weeks; therefore plasma exchange needs to be initiated with concomitant immunosuppressive therapy.

Patients may complain of paresthesias during the exchange due to citrate-induced hypocalcemia. Some can have nausea and vomiting due to alteration in electrolytes and fluid shifts.

(h) Intravenous Immunoglobulin (IVIg):

IVIg is usually a 4–6 h infusion for 5 days. It improves the weakness rapidly and lowers the AChR antibodies, often within 5 days of initiation of the infusion. Common side effects of IVIg infusion include headaches, myalgias, chills, chest discomfort, flu-like symptoms, urticaria, and pruritus of the palms. In patients with IgA deficiency, anaphylactic reactions may occur. Elderly patients with renal insufficiency have to be monitored for acute renal tubular necrosis, due to high concentration of sucrose in the IVIg product. Other uncommon side effects are aseptic meningitis, leukopenia, and DVT.

The choice between plasma exchange and IVIg lies in what is easily accessible, and the potential risks. In patients with renal issues, plasma exchange is better [23–25].

(i) Other options: Cyclophosphamide can be used in treatment resistant myasthenia gravis. The side effect profile includes alopecia, nausea, diarrhea, vomiting, hemorrhagic cystitis, and can cause infertility [26].

Rituximab, a monoclonal antibody against CD20 on the surface of B-cell has been used in some patients with limited results.

(j) Thymectomy: When initially performed, the mortality was about 80%, but with the recent advances, the mortality now has been negligible. This is mainly indicated for MG patients with thymoma. They improve if the surrounding thymus gland is also resected along with the thymoma [8].

Lambert–Eaton Syndrome

Lambert–Eaton myasthenic syndrome (LEMS) is a disorder of the peripheral cholinergic synapses characterized by proximal weakness and some autonomic dysfunction. In LEMS, antibodies are directed against the presynaptic voltage-gated Ca^{++} channels.

Epidemiology

LEMS is a rare disorder and found essentially only in adults. It is usually seen in smoking men >40 years. The incidence and prevalence of LEMS are significantly much lower than those of myasthenia. Paraneoplastic accounts for 50% of the LEMS cases, and about 80% of these occur in patients with small-cell lung carcinoma (SCLC). The other tumors implicated with LEMS are thymoma, lymphoma, renal cell cancer, and reproductive tract tumors; however, there is a strong suspicion of an underlying coexisting SCLC. Extrapulmonary primary small-cell carcinoma such as tongue, larynx, breast, pancreas, cervix, prostate, or skin (Merkel cell carcinoma) should also be considered in patients presenting with LEMS [27–32].

In idiopathic LEMS, the onset can vary from the very first decade to old age. The patients affected with idiopathic LEMS are nonsmokers, and often have a history of autoimmune diseases, either personally or in a family [33]. Females are more commonly affected in idiopathic LEMS.

What Causes Lambert–Eaton?

Lambert–Eaton myasthenic syndrome involves the production of IgG antibodies against the presynaptic P/Q voltage-gated calcium channels ($Ca_v2.1$), leading to a decreased release of calcium-dependent Ach from the presynaptic membrane. This decrement in the amount of Ach release will result in a reduced end-plate potential (EPP) below threshold on the postsynaptic membrane, thereby blocking the transmission at the NMJ [34].

The antigenic sites on the voltage-gated calcium channels bear a resemblance to the cell lines from small-cell lung carcinoma, and other neuroendocrine tumors. Glial nuclear antigen, a transcription factor spotted in patients with both SCLC and LEMS, but was absent in LEMS alone [8].

Clinical Features

The Course

LEMS presents months to years prior to the diagnosis of cancer. LEMS progresses quickly in the first year with a lower rate of remission, irrespective of the presence of cancer.

In patients with LEMS who are at a risk for SCLC, when the chest X-ray, sputum cytology, and CT come back negative, then the diagnostic yield for a neoplasm can be increased with a MRI/PET chest, bronchoscopy with transbronchial biopsy, thoracoscopy or transesophageal ultrasound. If the chest workup is negative, then searching for an extrapulmonary small-cell carcinoma is necessary. It is noted that SCLC responds well to treatment in patients who present with LEMS, may be due to the early diagnosis of the symptoms. Many of the times, the strength improves post treatment of the underlying malignancy [35, 36].

The Symptoms and Signs

The most common presenting symptoms of LEMS is weakness, subacute progressive fatigue, and unanticipated falls. The characteristic of the weakness in LEMS is that intensifies with exercise and transiently alleviates with rest. The weakness has a pattern, with symptoms typically starting in the hip flexors and other proximal lower limb muscles. Most of the patients complain of difficulty in climbing stairs, or arising from a chair. Proximal muscles of the upper limb and the interossei of the hand are affected sometimes. Cranial muscle involvement (ptosis, dysphagia, dysarthria, facial weakness, difficulty chewing) is milder in comparison to myasthenia gravis. Fasciculations, cramps, and atrophy are rare. In paraneoplastic LEMS, sometimes patients may experience pain in the hip and posterior thigh.

Other sensory symptoms almost never present, unless there is a paraneoplastic manifestation of radiculoplexopathy or neuropathy. Deep tendon reflexes are present early in the disease, but are typically reduced or absent. The easier bedside test is to demonstrate the facilitation of the reflex after a spell of brief exercise.

In patients with SCLC and LEMS, symptoms of hemoptysis and chest pain are uncommon. In patients with idiopathic LEMS, symptoms of autoimmune disorders like pernicious anemia, hyperthyroidism, or hypothyroidism are common [35, 36].

In about 80% of the LEMS patients, autonomic dysfunction results in orthostatic hypotension, urinary retention, gastrointestinal dysmotility, slow pupillary reflexes, xerostomia, and impotence [33]. Autoimmune gastroparesis can present with anorexia and weight loss, and suggests an underlying malignancy.

Diagnosis

(a) Clinical: LEMS is suspected in a patient with weakness that worsens with exertion. The clinical features for the diagnosis of LEMS have been described in the section above.
(b) Laboratory and Electrodiagnostic studies: Antibodies against the P/Q voltage-gated calcium channels ($Ca_v2.1$) are present in >90% of non-immunosuppressed LEMS patients [37]. N-type ($Ca_v2.2$) calcium channel antibodies are seen in about 75% of LEMS patients with lung cancer, and at 40% without cancer risks [37].

P/Q type and N-type antibodies also serve as serological markers of paraneoplastic neurological disorders other than LEMS, associated with SCLC, breast and ovarian carcinoma. In about 13% of patients with LEMS, nicotinic AChR antibodies can be seen [36, 38, 39].

The characteristic electrodiagnostic features in LEMS are the reduced CMAP amplitude, and this decrement is more prominent with slow RNS, and the facilitation of >200% is noticed following brief exercise, or a high frequency

RNS due to increase in the number of ACh quanta. Needle EMG shows varying low-amplitude MUP.

Treatment

Treating LEMS with drugs facilitating the release of ACh, like 3,4-diaminopyridine has shown both clinical and electrophysiologic improvement. Pyridostigmine bromide and 3,4-diaminopyridine when used in combination improves strength, but 3,4-diaminopyridine is not currently approved by the U.S. Food and Drug Administration (FDA) [8].

Other therapeutic options like steroids, plasma exchange, IVIg, and immunosuppressive agents.

(a) Tumor therapy: Treating the tumor will actually ameliorate the symptoms of LEMS. When the cancer is SCLC, treatment with chemotherapy and radiation usually cures the LEMS most of the times. But patients with post tumor therapy will still need symptomatic treatment or immunotherapy [40].
(b) Cholinesterase Inhibitors:

   In order to have a beneficial effect, cholinesterase inhibitors need to be combined with medications that raise the ACh level, like guanidine or 3,4-diaminopyridine.

   Guanidine inhibits the calcium uptake, thereby increasing the intracellular calcium in the nerve terminal, and that releases more quanta of Ach [41]. Guanidine is effective when the dose is limited, and used in combination with pyridostigmine [42, 43]. Side effects of guanidine include renal and hematopoietic toxicity [44, 45].

   3,4-diaminopyridine acts by blocking K_v channels within the nerve terminal, extending the action potential through enhancing the Ca^{++} entry. Clinically the strength improves, and electrodiagnostically there is an elevation in the amplitude, along with a reduced CMAP decrement. Single-fiber EMG shows reduced to minimal jitter and blocking [46, 47]. It can cause light-headedness, headache, seizures, insomnia, and sometimes cardiac arrhythmia. This is the reason patients need a screening EKG and EEG to rule out arrhythmias and seizures [48].
(c) Immunotherapy: It is usually indicated in patients who fail to improve post tumor therapy, or symptomatic therapy. IVIg, corticosteroids, and plasmapheresis have shown some benefit. Plasmapheresis is generally reserved for respiratory insufficiency. Oral corticosteroids do show some improvement in strength, but lesser than in myasthenia gravis [35, 36].

Botulism

Botulinum toxin through its actions on the presynaptic membrane causes a near total paralysis of both nicotinic and muscarinic cholinergic transmission. The heavy chain especially mediates binding of the toxin to the motor nerve terminals and also aids the light chain to be translocated into the cytoplasm. This light chain cleaves the synaptic vesicle components based on the toxin serotype. Toxins B,G, and F cleave synaptobrevin, whereas A and E cleave SNAP-25, along with Type B for synaptotagmin. All these interfere with the calcium-dependent intracellular cascade responsible for ACh release.

Clostridium botulinum spores contaminate foods and produce A, B, F, and G. Type A causes the maximum damage.

Botulism can be classified under four clinical forms, depending on the mode of entry: Food-borne botulism—most common, wound botulism, infant botulism, and iatrogenic botulism [8].

Clinical Features

The most common form of the disease results from ingestion of foods contaminated with spores. It is noted that not all who ingest the contaminated food are symptomatic. Typically,

nausea and vomiting are the very first symptoms, with neuromuscular manifestations showing up 12–36 h post exposure.

Ptosis, dysphagia, dysarthria, and blurred vision with mydriatic pupils that react poorly to light are the usual features. The weakness descends progressively over 4–5 days before plateauing, but the respiratory paralysis is rapid. Dysautonomic manifestations like dry mouth, urinary retention, constipation, and cardiovascular instability [49].

Wound botulism presents the same way as classical botulism, but the mode of entry is by the contamination of the wound with C. botulinum spores. This form of botulism is pretty rare [50].

Infantile botulism usually affects infants younger than 6 months. Honey is the most common source of contamination, from where the toxin is consumed. Symptoms of weakness typically tend to descend with cranial, axial, and limb muscle involvement, besides reduced spontaneous movements, lethargy, poor suck, and constipation. These symptoms most commonly occur between 2 and 8 months of age. The level of respiratory compromise is very severe, with most of them requiring mechanical ventilation [51].

Some cases of botulism happen without any apparent identifiable cause, and such cases are known as hidden botulism [52, 53]. Sometimes, *C. botulinum* can grow in the intestine, post-surgery from antibiotic therapy or gastric achlorhydria [54].

How to Diagnose Botulism?
(a) Clinical: Botulism presents with the features as described above. The features of botulism and LEMS are similar, but the most important differentiating factor is the acuity of the presentation. Botulism is acute and severe, where LEMS is more gradual [8].

(b) Laboratory and Electrodiagnostic: In suspected botulism patients, the toxin needs to be identified from the serum, stool, or the residual food samples. The Center for Disease Control and Prevention (CDC) runs a 24 h emergency helpline to guide with the proper collection of the samples and the treatment options. Besides the toxin, C. botulinum per se should be looked for in the stools in cases of infantile botulism [8].

Electrophysiologically, the baseline CMAP is of low amplitude, due to inadequate release of ACh quanta.

Rapid repetitive nerve stimulation (RNS) is the key for presynaptic neuromuscular junction disorders like LEMS and botulism. There is an increment of up to 200% in the evoked response on rapid RNS at 20–50 Hz or after exercise in botulism. The conventional needle EMG can be normal or may show short duration polyphasic MUAP, and some fibrillations.

TREATMENT: Botulism usually needs emergency hospitalization. CDC recommends using the antitoxin, and guanidine as therapy for botulism. As mentioned earlier in this chapter, guanidine helps in the neurotransmission by promoting the release of ACh from the presynaptic terminal. Always watch out for the side effects from antitoxin—serum sickness or anaphylaxis; and guanidine—bone marrow suppression.

In a few patients, intravenous edrophonium chloride improves the ptosis, but the effect is not sustained. Infantile botulism is a medical emergency and invariably needs respiratory support with mechanical ventilation. It is imperative to avoid honey in babies under the age of 1 year. In order to attenuate the time on the ventilator and indirectly the stay in the hospital, botulinum immune globulin (BIG) is sometimes administered [8].

Sleep Disorders in NMJ

Sleep disorders are pretty common in patients with neuromuscular junction disorders, and in neuromuscular diseases in general. The most common sleep disorder in neuromuscular diseases is sleep-disordered breathing (SDB) [55]. Sleep-disordered breathing includes obstructive sleep apnea (OSA), central sleep apnea, and mixed sleep apnea showing features of both central and obstructive.

SDB symptoms usually progress gradually, most often times, patients being unaware of it most of the times. It is a significant cause of morbidity and mortality among patients with neuromuscular diseases [55]. Therefore, an early diagnosis and treatment of SDB can lead to a better quality of life, and thus prolonging the survival in patients with neuromuscular diseases.

Symptoms like excessive daytime sleepiness, fatigue, nocturnal abnormal movements, nocturnal restlessness, unexplained arousals from sleep, cognitive dysfunction, dyspnea, orthopnea, morning headaches, failure to thrive, and declining grades in the pediatric population should indicate the possibility of sleep-disordered breathing in these patients [55].

Though these symptoms point towards SDB, it is not uncommon to have patients not manifest these symptoms in spite of having a significant SDB.

Excessive daytime sleepiness (EDS), unexplained frequent arousals from sleep with choking/gasping, and fatigue increase the suspicion for obstructive sleep apnea (OSA). Epworth Sleepiness Scale (ESS) scoring on a scale of 0–24 is a good measure of excessive daytime sleepiness, with scores >10 pointing towards pathological hypersomnolence. However, in patients with neuromuscular diseases, ESS score has a poor to no correlation with the degree of nocturnal hypoxia [56]. Nocturnal hypoxia leading to nocturnal shortness of breath and orthopnea is a sign of early respiratory hypoventilation due to neuromuscular weakness [56]. Morning headaches, cognitive impairment, dream-enactment behaviors, and excessive movements in sleep are some of the additional symptoms that can raise a suspicion of sleep-disordered breathing [57].

Other sleep disorders associated with neuromuscular diseases are restless legs syndrome (RLS), daytime sleepiness, limb movement disorder, etc.

In this section of the chapter, we are going to address the sleep disorders commonly seen in neuromuscular junction disorders like myasthenia gravis, Lambert–Eaton syndrome, and botulism.

Sleep Issues in Myasthenia gravis (MG)

Myasthenia gravis is an autoimmune neuromuscular junction disorder characterized by fatigability and episodic weakness of the skeletal muscles. Repetitive voluntary muscles usage results in weakness, and rest restores normalcy. The most commonly encountered sleep disorder in MG is sleep-disordered breathing (SDB) [58].

Sleep-Disordered Breathing (SDB)

Various factors play a role in sleep-disordered breathing in myasthenic patients.

It is possibly due to the combination of

(a) Respiratory muscle weakness leading to alveolar hypoventilation.
(b) Raised upper airway resistance owing to pharyngeal dilator muscle hypotonia [55].

About 40–60% of patients with stable myasthenia gravis have sleep-disordered breathing, a majority of which is central sleep apneas and hypopneas, and occurs in the REM sleep [59]. Since MG is a fairly unstable disease in terms of presentation, there is a lot of variability in the associated sleep disorders. Respiratory weakness is seen in about 30% of the myasthenic patients, typically late in the disease and there is a weak correlation with the severity of MG [60]. Thus, a patient with mild MG can have clinically severe ventilatory issues requiring mechanical ventilation, due to oropharyngeal, diaphragmatic, and intercostal muscle weakness.

There have been multiple studies looking into the association between sleep-disordered breathing and myasthenia gravis. In 1976, Papazian first demonstrated that myasthenic patients showed altered REM sleep due to disturbance in the acetylcholine mechanism in the central nervous system [61]. This was followed up with a study by Mennuni et al., who reiterated that patients with MG had altered REM sleep (shorter REM sleep) due to fatigability inside the REM periods [62]. In contrast to this observation, Stepansky et al. conducted a study on 19 middle-aged MG patients, and disproved the hypothesis of decreased REM sleep duration [63].

Amino et al. suggested that sleep apnea is a possible clinical manifestation of a nocturnal dysfunction of both central and peripheral cholinergic systems, and that is the reason why both central and obstructive sleep apnea occur in MG [64]. But, according to the study by Stepansky et al., it was suggested that a disturbance of the central cholinergic system was "highly unlikely" as the REM sleep was unaffected in MG [63]. In summary, sleep disturbances in MG most likely originate in the peripheral system rather than the central, and the resultant hypoxia may worsen during sleep, especially REM sleep.

In patients with myasthenia gravis, prevalence of obstructive sleep apnea was noted to be much higher in comparison to general population [65], and the number of awakenings due to the obstructive events was also noted to be higher in patients with MG [66].

And that is why, in many of the studies involving myasthenia gravis patients, excessive daytime sleepiness was reported as high due to sleep fragmentation. Excessive daytime sleepiness (EDS) is one of the classical manifestations of sleep-disordered breathing, along with snoring, choking, gasping events, and fatigue. EDS can be demonstrated on the Epworth Sleepiness Scale (ESS). In a study by Quera-Salva et al., one-third of the patients with MG checked excessive daytime sleepiness on the ESS [67].

The other significant symptom that patients with MG present is fatigue. MG is characterized by progressive fatigability, and it was demonstrated that patients with MG have higher levels of fatigue scores, even among those in complete remission [68]. Kassardjian et al. suggested that the neuromuscular fatigue in myasthenic patients improves with daytime naps, with naps as short as 5 min [69].

But when dealing with fatigue in myasthenic patients, it is imperative to rule out obstructive sleep apnea as a causal factor for the fatigue; this would avoid unnecessary increments in the corticosteroid therapy for myasthenic fatigue.

Restless Legs Syndrome (RLS)/Willis Ekbom Disease

Despite its name, this disorder is not always confined to legs.

Diagnosing restless legs syndrome is essentially clinical and is defined by the presence of four key criteria: unpleasant sensation in the legs, causing an urge to move them; circadian pattern with symptoms worse in the evening and night; symptoms induced by rest; and activity causing a relief [70]. Other clinical features suggestive for RLS include the tendency for symptoms to gradually worsen with age, improvement with dopaminergic treatments, periodic limb movements while asleep (PLMS), and a positive family history [71]. Besides these, there are specific criteria for special groups (elderly and children).

The most common conditions associated with RLS include pregnancy, systemic iron deficiency, renal failure, neuropathy, myelinopathy, multiple sclerosis, and possibly Parkinson disease and essential tremor [71].

Restless legs syndrome and its association with myasthenia gravis was studied by Siemenski et al. Using a questionnaire, they noticed that about 43% of the MG patients had restless legs syndrome, and more than half of this population considered RLS as a troublesome health issue [72]. In a recently concluded study by Wang et al., about one-fourth of the patients with myasthenia complained of restless legs. Management of RLS in myasthenia gravis is no different from restless legs in the general population, with dopamine agonists being the most widely accepted and investigated treatment option. Other treatments include alpha-2 delta blockers, opioids, and iron. Certain alpha-2 delta blockers like gabapentin encarbil are used to counter augmentation in patients with RLS [71].

Sleep Issues in Lambert–Eaton Myasthenic Syndrome

LEMS is a less common disorder of the neuromuscular junction than myasthenia gravis. This is an autoimmune condition, wherein antibodies are formed against the voltage-gated calcium channels in the presynaptic junction. This interrupts the neurotransmission due to reduced release of ACh quanta. Most commonly it is associated with small-cell lung cancer (SCLC), and is characterized by proximal muscle weakness, areflexia, dysautonomia, and post-tetanic potentiation on electrophysiological studies [73].

Since the presentation is similar to myasthenia in terms of respiratory weakness, sleep-disordered breathing and other sleep disorders can occur in LEMS. Further studies are needed to analyze the prevalence and severity of these sleep-related disorders in LEMS.

Diagnosis of Sleep Issues in NMJ Disorders

Sleep-disordered breathing or sleep-related breathing disorder is very common in neuromuscular diseases and is usually seen before the onset of respiratory compromise in these patients. Besides the clinical symptoms of snoring, choking or gasping, fatigue and daytime sleepiness; simple office-based questionnaires and tests have been developed to predict the presence of sleep dysfunction in neuromuscular diseases. Steier et al. developed the Sleep-Disordered Breathing in Neuromuscular Disease Questionnaire (SINQ-5). This questionnaire comprises five questions related to sleep, posture, and breathlessness; and is scored on a scale of 0–10, with lower scores implying fewer symptoms [74]. Patients can be screened with other screening tools like Epworth Sleepiness Scale (ESS),

Pittsburgh Sleep Quality Index (PQSI), and STOP-BANG. Single-breath test is a simple test to detect the vital capacity by asking the patient to take a maximum inspiratory breath and count. Normally, the count can go up to 50 on the maximum inspiratory breath, but patients with impaired vital capacity can count until 15 or less.

Polysomnography is the gold standard test to diagnose sleep-disordered breathing, and other alterations in sleep such as insomnia, periodic limb movement disorder, and reduced sleep efficiency. If there is a suspicion of an associated narcolepsy, a multiple sleep latency test (MSLT) is useful. Assessing the arterial blood gases, gas exchange, and the lung volumes can be used as an adjunct to the conventional polysomnogram.

Iron deficiency is a strong association with RLS, and all RLS patients should be tested for it. It is advisable to get iron levels, transferrin saturation, ferritin levels, and the total iron binding capacity; as ferritin is a marker of inflammation, and can be falsely elevated [55].

Treatment for Sleep Issues in NMJ Disorders

For patients with sleep-related breathing disorders, non-invasive ventilation is the standard of treatment. Non-invasive positive pressure ventilation (NPPV) is the better option, when there is an underlying hypoventilation component. Bilevel positive pressure ventilation along with supplemental oxygen is tolerated well in patients with neuromuscular disease. For patients with obstructive sleep apnea, continuous positive airway pressure (CPAP) has shown maximum benefits, by not only correcting the apneas, but also the symptoms of ocular myasthenia. The possible explanation for the correlation between SDB and ocular MG is a decreased acetylcholine sensitivity to the acetylcholine receptor as a result of hypoxia induced lowered ATP levels. That's why if given CPAP, it would correct the hypercapnia and improve both the symptoms of SDB and ocular MG [75].

For myasthenic patients, even when adequately treated to the point of being symptom free during the day, it is still possible for them to have sleep-disordered breathing at night. Besides the conventional therapy for SDB in MG, a study demonstrated that thymectomy may actually lower the prevalence of SDB in MG, as the respiratory events in sleep are likely due to the changes in activity at the neuromuscular junction [64]. Other therapeutic options like plasmapheresis have not shown any clinical benefit on the sleep issues, despite showing clinical improvement in terms of weakness, lower myasthenia gravis score, and anti-AChR antibody testing.

For MG patients with restless legs syndrome, besides the commonly used pharmacotherapy with dopaminergic agonists, benzodiazepines, clonidine, gabapentin, and pregabalin, it is important to supplement iron, as many of these patients have an associated iron deficiency anemia [71].

Key Points

1. Myasthenia gravis is an autoimmune disease with fluctuating symptoms. The autoantibodies are directed against the acetylcholine receptors in the neuromuscular junction. Respiratory muscle involvement as the first sign of the disease is usually rare.
2. Myasthenic crisis (MC) can be provoked by various factors like a surgical procedure, or a respiratory infection, and sometimes can occur without any provocation. It is a complication of MG causing respiratory compromise and failure, and would need intubation and assisted ventilation.
3. About 40–60% of patients with stable myasthenia gravis have sleep-disordered breathing.
4. Lambert–Eaton myasthenic syndrome (LEMS) is characterized by antibodies that are directed against the presynaptic voltage-gated Ca^{++} channels.
5. LEMS is most commonly associated with small-cell lung cancer (SCLC) and is characterized by proximal muscle weakness, areflexia, dysautonomia, and post-tetanic potentiation on electrophysiological studies.
6. Botulinum toxin through its actions on the presynaptic membrane causes a near total paralysis of both nicotinic and muscarinic cholinergic transmission.
7. The most common conditions associated with RLS include pregnancy, systemic iron deficiency, renal failure, and neuropathy.

References

1. Kandel E, Schwartz J, Jessell T. Principles of neural science. 4th ed. New York: McGraw-Hill; 2000.
2. Magleby KI. Neuromuscular transmission. In: The anatomy, physiology, and biochemistry of muscle (Chapter 13). p. 393–418.
3. Adrian RH. The effect of internal and external potassium concentration on the membrane potential of frog muscle. J Physiol. 1956;133:631–58.
4. Rowland LP, Merritt HH. Merritt's neurology. Philadelphia: Lippincott Williams & Wilkins; 2005.
5. Somnier FE, Keiding N, Paulson OB. Epidemiology of myasthenia gravis in Denmark. A longitudinal and comprehensive population survey. Arch Neurol. 1991;48:733–9.
6. Phillips LH, Torner JC, Anderson MS, Cox GM. The epidemiology of myasthenia gravis in central and western Virginia. Neurology. 1992;42:1888–93.
7. Vincent A, McConville J, Farrugia ME, Newsom-Davis J. Seronegative myasthenia gravis. Semin Neurol. 2004;24:125–33.
8. Ulane CM, Lewis PR. Merritt's neurology. Philadelphia: Lippincott Williams & Wilkins; 2015.
9. Cohen MS, Younger D. Aspects of the natural history of myasthenia gravis: crisis and death. Ann N Y Acad Sci. 1981;377:670–7.
10. Wittbrodt ET. Drugs and myasthenia gravis. An update. Arch Intern Med. 1997;157:399–408.
11. Plauché WC. Myasthenia gravis in pregnancy: an update. Am J Obstet Gynecol. 1979;135:691–7.

12. Crain SM, Bornstein MB, Lennon VA. Depression of complex bioelectric discharges in cultured cerebral tissue cultures by thermolabile dependent serum factors. Exp Neurol. 1975;49:330–5.
13. Kuks JBM. Clinical presentation and epidemiology of myasthenia gravis. Myasthenia gravis and related disorders. New York: Springer; 2008. https://doi.org/10.1007/978-1-59745-156-7_5.
14. Oosterhuis HJGH. Myasthenia gravis. Edinburgh: Churchill Livingstone; 1984.
15. Palace J, Newsom-Davis J, Lecky BA. Randomized doubleblind trial of prednisolone alone or with azathioprine in myasthenia gravis. Myasthenia gravis study group. Neurology. 1998;50(6):1778–83.
16. Myasthenia Gravis Clinical Study Group. A randomised clinical trial comparing prednisone and azathioprine in myasthenia gravis. Results of the second interim analysis. J Neurol Neurosurg Psychiatry. 1993;56(11):1157–63.
17. Tindall RS, Rollins JA, Phillips JT, et al. Preliminary results of a double-blind, randomized, placebo controlled trial of cyclosporine in myasthenia gravis. N Engl J Med. 1987;316(12):719–24. https://doi.org/10.1056/NEJM198703193161205.
18. Tindall RS, Phillips JT, Rollins JA, et al. A clinical therapeutic trial of cyclosporine in myasthenia gravis. Ann N Y Acad Sci. 1993;681:539–51.
19. Meriggioli MN, Ciafaloni E, Al-Hayk KA, et al. Mycophenolate mofetil for myasthenia gravis: an analysis of efficacy, safety, and tolerability. Neurology. 2003;61(10):1438–40.
20. Sanders DB, Hart IK, Mantegazza R, et al. An international, phase III, randomized trial of mycophenolate mofetil in myasthenia gravis. Neurology. 2008;71(6):400–6. https://doi.org/10.1212/01.wnl.0000312374.95186.cc.
21. Muscle Study Group. A trial of mycophenolate mofetil with prednisone as initial immunotherapy in myasthenia gravis. Neurology. 2008;71(6):394–9. https://doi.org/10.1212/01.wnl.0000312373.67493.7f.
22. Nagane Y, Utsugisawa K, Obara D, et al. Efficacy of lowdose FK506 in the treatment of myasthenia gravis—a randomized pilot study. Eur Neurol. 2005;53(3):146–50. https://doi.org/10.1159/000085833.
23. Gajdos P, Tranchant C, Clair B, et al. Treatment of myasthenia gravis exacerbation with intravenous immunoglobulin: a randomized double-blind clinical trial. Arch Neurol. 2005;62(11):1689–93. https://doi.org/10.1001/archneur.62.11.1689.
24. Zinman L, Ng E, Bril V. IV immunoglobulin in patients with myasthenia gravis: a randomized controlled trial. Neurology. 2007;68(11):837–41. https://doi.org/10.1212/01.wnl.0000256698.69121.45.
25. Barth D, Nabavi Nouri M, Ng E, et al. Comparison of IVIg and PLEX in patients with myasthenia gravis. Neurology. 2011;76(23):2017–23. https://doi.org/10.1212/WNL.0b013e31821e5505.
26. De Feo LG, Schottlender J, Martelli NA, et al. Use of intravenous pulsed cyclophosphamide in severe, generalized myasthenia gravis. Muscle Nerve. 2002;26(1):31–6. https://doi.org/10.1002/mus.10133.
27. Gutmann L, Phillips LH, Gutmann L. Trends in the association of Lambert-Eaton myasthenic syndrome with carcinoma. Neurology. 1992;42:848–50.
28. Argov Z, Shapira Y, Averbuch-Heller L, Wirguin I. Lambert-Eaton myasthenic syndrome (LES) in association with lymphoproliferative disorders. Muscle Nerve. 1995;18:715–9.
29. Burns TM, Juel VC, Sanders DB, Phillips LH. Neuroendocrine lung tumors and disorders of the neuromuscular junction. Neurology. 1999;52:1490–1.
30. Collins DR, Connolly S, Burns M, Offiah L, Grainger R, Walsh JB. Lambert-Eaton myasthenic syndrome in association with transitional cell carcinoma: a previously unrecognized association. Urology. 1999;54:162.
31. Dalmau J, Gultekin HS, Posner JB. Paraneoplastic neurologic syndromes: pathogenesis and physiopathology. Brain Pathol. 1999;9:275–84.
32. Oyaizu T, Okada Y, Sagawa M, Yamakawa K, Kuroda H, Fujihara K, Itoyama Y, Tanita T, Motomura M, Kondo T. Lambert-Eaton myasthenic syndrome associated with an anterior mediastinal small cell carcinoma. J Thorac Cardiovasc Surg. 2001;121:1005–6.

33. O'Neill JH, Murray NM, Newsom-Davis J. The Lambert-Eaton myasthenic syndrome. A review of 50 cases. Brain. 1988;111:577–96.
34. Waterman SA, Lang B, Newsom-Davis J. Effect of Lambert-Eaton myasthenic syndrome antibodies on autonomic neurons in the mouse. Ann Neurol. 1997;42:147–56.
35. Harper CM. Electrodiagnosis of endplate disease. In: Engel AG, editor. Myasthenia gravis and myasthenic syndromes. New York: Oxford Press; 1999. p. 65–86.
36. Lennon VA. Serological diagnosis of myasthenia gravis and the Lambert-Eaton myasthenic syndrome. In: Lisak R, editor. Handbook of myasthenia gravis, chapter 7. New York: Marcel Dekker; 1994. p. 149–64.
37. Lennon VA, Kryzer TJ, Greismann GE, O'Suilleabhain PE, Windebank AJ, Woppmann A, Miljanich GP, Lambert E. Calcium channel antibodies in the Lambert-Eaton myasthenic syndrome and other paraneoplastic syndromes. N Engl J Med. 1995;332:1467–74.
38. Vernino S, Adamski J, Kryzer TJ, Lennon VA. Neuronal nicotinic AChR antibody in subacute autonomic neuropathy and cancer-related syndromes. Neurology. 1998;50:1806–13.
39. Lennon VA. Serologic profile of myasthenia gravis and distinction from Lambert-Eaton myasthenic syndrome. Neurology. 1997;48(Suppl 5):S23–7.
40. Maddison P, Newsom-Davis J, Mills KR, Souhami RL. Favorable prognosis in Lambert-Eaton myasthenic syndrome and small-cell lung carcinoma. Lancet. 1999;353:117–8.
41. Kamenskaya MA, Elmqvist D, Thesleff S. Guanidine and neuromuscular transmission. II. Effect on transmitter release in response to repetitive nerve stimulation. Arch Neurol. 1975;32:510–8.
42. Oh SJ, Kim DS, Head TC, Claussen GC. Low dose guanidine and pyridostigmine: relatively safe and effective longterm symptomatic therapy in Lambert-Eaton myasthenic syndrome. Muscle Nerve. 1997;20:1146–52.
43. Silbert PL, Hankey GJ, Barr AL. Successful alternate day guanidine therapy following guanidine-induced neutropenia in the Lambert-Eaton myasthenic syndrome. Muscle Nerve. 1990;13:360–1.
44. Cherington M. Guanidine and germine in Eaton-Lambert syndrome. Neurology. 1976;26:944–6.
45. Blumhardt LD, Joekes AM, Marshall J, Philalithis PE. Guanidine treatment and impaired renal function in the Eaton-Lambert syndrome. Br Med J. 1977;1:946–7.
46. Harper CM, McEvoy KM, Windebank AJ, Daube JR. Effect of 3,4-diaminopyridine on neuromuscular transmission in patients with Lambert-Eaton myasthenic syndrome. Electroencephalogr Clin Neurophysiol. 1990;75:557.
47. Kim DS, Claussen GC, Oh SJ. Single-fiber electromyography improvement with 3,4-diaminopyridine in Lambert-Eaton myasthenic syndrome. Muscle Nerve. 1998;21:1107–8.
48. Boerma CE, Rommes JH, van Leeuwen RB, Bakker J. Cardiac arrest following an iatrogenic 3,4-diaminopyridine intoxication in a patient with Lambert-Eaton myasthenic syndrome. Clin Toxicol. 1995;33:249–51.
49. Sanders D, Howard F Jr. Disorders of neuromuscular transmission. In: Bradley W, Daroff R, Fenichel G, Marsden C, editors. Neurology in clinical practice. Boston: Butterworth Heinemann; 2000. p. 2167–85.
50. MacDonald KL, Rutherford SM, Friedman SM, Dieter JA, Kaye BR, McKinley GF, Tenney JH, Cohen ML. Botulism and botulism-like illness in chronic drug users. Ann Intern Med. 1985;102:616–8.
51. Pickett J, Berg B, Chaplin E, Brunstetter-Shafer M. Syndrome of botulism in infancy: clinical and electrophysiologic study. N Engl J Med. 1976;295:770–92.
52. Chia JK, Clark JB, Ryan CA, Pollack M. Botulism in an adult associated with food-borne intestinal infection with Clostridium botulinum. N Engl J Med. 1986;315:239–41.
53. Dowell VR Jr, McCroskey LM, Hatheway CL, Lombard GL, Hughes JM, Merson MH. Coproexamination for botulinal toxin and clostridium botulinum. A new procedure for laboratory diagnosis of botulism. JAMA. 1977;238:1829–32.
54. Griffin PM, Hatheway CL, Rosenbaum RB, Sokolow R. Endogenous antibody production to botulinum toxin in an adult with intestinal colonization botulism and underlying Crohn's disease. J Infect Dis. 1997;175:633–7.

55. Bhat S, Gupta D, Chokroverty S. Sleep disorders in neuromuscular diseases. Neurol Clin. 2012;30:1359–87.
56. Furuta H, Kaneda R, Kosaka K, et al. Epworth sleepiness scale and sleep studies in patients with obstructive sleep apnea syndrome. Psychiatry Clin Neurosci. 1999;53(2):301.
57. Chokroverty S. Sleep and breathing in neuromuscular disorders. Handb Clin Neurol. 2011;99:1087–108.
58. Fernandes Oliveira E, Nacif SR, Alves Pereira N, et al. Sleep disorders in patients with myasthenia gravis: a systematic review. J Phys Ther Sci. 2015;27(6):2013–8. https://doi.org/10.1589/jpts.27.2013.
59. Manni R, Piccolo G, Sartori I, et al. Breathing during sleep in myasthenia gravis. Ital J Neurol Sci. 1995;16(9):589–94.
60. Fermin AM, Afzal U, Culebras A. Sleep in neuromuscular diseases. Sleep Med Clin. 2016;11(1):53–64. Online publication date: 1-Mar-2016.
61. Papazian O. Rapid eye movement sleep alterations in myasthenia gravis. Neurology. 1976;26:311–6.
62. Mennuni G, Morante MT, Di Meo L, et al. [Myasthenia and sleep]. Schweiz Arch Neurol Neurochir Psychiatr. 1983;133:193–203.
63. Stepansky R, Weber G, Zeitlhofer J. Sleep apnea and cognitive dysfunction in myasthenia gravis. Acta Med Austriaca. 1997;24:128–31.
64. Amino A, Shiozawa Z, Nagasaka T, et al. Sleep apnoea in well-controlled myasthenia gravis and the effect of thymectomy. J Neurol. 1998;245:77–80.
65. Nicolle MW, Rask S, Koopman WJ, et al. Sleep apnea in patients with myasthenia gravis. Neurology. 2006;67:140–2.
66. Happe S, Klösch G, Zeitlhofer J. Perception of dreams and subjective sleep quality in patients with myasthenia gravis. Neuropsychobiology. 2004;50:21–7.
67. Quera-Salva MA, Guilleminault C, Chevret S, et al. Breathing disorders during sleep in myasthenia gravis. Ann Neurol. 1992;31:86–92.
68. Elsais A, Wyller VB, Loge JH, et al. Fatigue in myasthenia gravis: is it more than muscular weakness? BMC Neurol. 2013;13:132.
69. Kassardjian CD, Murray BJ, Kokokyi S, et al. Effects of napping on neuromuscular fatigue in myasthenia gravis. Muscle Nerve. 2013;48:816–8.
70. Allen RP, Picchietti D, Hening WA, et al. Restless legs syndrome: diagnostic criteria, special considerations, and epidemiology A report from the restless legs syndrome diagnosis and epidemiology workshop at the National Institutes of Health. Sleep Med. 2003;42(2):101–19.
71. Ondo WG. Restless legs syndrome. Neurol Clin. 2009;27(3):779–99.
72. Sieminski M, Bilińska M, Nyka WM. Increased frequency of restless legs syndrome in myasthenia gravis. Eur Neurol. 2012;68:166–70.
73. Kimura J. Electrodiagnosis in diseases of the nerve and muscle, principles and practice. 3rd ed. Oxford: New York; 2001.
74. Steier J, Jolley CJ, Seymour J, et al. Screening for sleep-disordered breathing in neuromuscular disease using a questionnaire for symptoms associated with diaphragm paralysis. Eur Respir J. 2011;37(2):400–5.
75. Naseer S, Kolade VO, Idrees S, et al. Improvement in ocular myasthenia gravis during CPAP therapy for sleep apnea. Tenn Med. 2012;105(9):33–4.

Sleep Disorders in Peripheral Neuropathy

6

Satish Bokka, Raghav Govindarajan, and Nakul Katyal

Recent studies have made it very clear that sleep disturbances (insomnia, sleep apnea, periodic limb movement disorder) have a major impact on health and quality of life. These sleep issues are frequently overlooked in regular medical interviews. Sleep issues are especially debilitating in patients with peripheral neuropathy.

Several scales are used to detect sleep issues in patients with neuropathy. Some of them are DSIS (Daily Sleep Interference Scale), Epworth Sleepiness Scale, MOS (Medical Outcomes Study) sleep scale, Pittsburgh Sleep Quality Index, etc. Among those DSIS is more reliable and has good validity. It was developed particularly to quantify sleep disturbances due to pain. Patients were asked upon awakening about sleep interference due to pain on daily basis in order to minimize the recall bias. The DSIS is brief and can be easily incorporated into daily diaries. The DSIS has been recently used to assess sleep issues in diabetic peripheral neuropathy and postherpetic neuropathy patients [1].

The association of sleep issues and neuropathy is complex and a detailed description is beyond the scope of this book. In the next few paragraphs, we have briefly discussed sleep issues in five main conditions, namely Charcot–Marie–Tooth disease, diabetic neuropathy, multifocal neuropathy with conduction block, spinocerebellar ataxia, and association between restless legs syndrome and neuropathies.

In Charcot–Marie–Tooth (CMT) patients, both pharyngeal and laryngeal neuropathy can lead to severe sleep apnea. These neuropathies interfere with functional

---

S. Bokka, M.D.
Department of Neurology, University of Louisville School of Medicine, Louisville, KY, USA
e-mail: skbokk01@Louisville.edu

R. Govindarajan, M.D., F.A.A.N. (✉)
Department of Neurology, University of Missouri, Columbia, MO, USA
e-mail: govindarajanr@health.missouri.edu

N. Katyal, M.D.
University of Missouri, Columbia, MO, USA

status of pharyngeal group of muscles and those local reflexes preventing the upper airway collapse during inspiration. The hypoglossal nerve plays a significant role in motor control of pharyngeal musculature and is involved in upper airway protective reflexes. So both hypoglossal dysfunction and pharyngeal neuropathy are associated with OSA [2]. Some patients also have vocal cord palsy and phrenic neuropathy that affects the diaphragm functional ability and leads to hypoventilation. The severity of sleep apnea is directly proportional to the severity of peripheral neuropathy [2]. CMAP (compound muscle action potential) amplitude of median nerve was inversely correlated with apnea-hypopnea index. There was no relation between nerve conduction velocity and sleep apnea. Male family members had more severe neuropathy than women, probable explanation for that was progesterone dependent increase in genioglossus muscle activity while awake and continue during sleep. Progesterone also promotes myelin formation in peripheral nerves. Other risk factors for severe neuropathy in CMT patients is high body mass index and old age [3].

Half of all cases of apnea in CMT patients were due to central sleep apnea. Increased sensitivity to carbon dioxide, chemosensitivity and ventilator response to carbon dioxide, reduced $PaCO_2$ in patients with CMT are possible predictive values for central apnea [4]. In patients with hereditary sensory motor neuropathy who present with symptoms of nocturnal hypoventilation and unexplained cardiac failure, we should suspect the possibility of diaphragmatic weakness. The diagnosis is confirmed by measuring FVC, abdominal movements during inspiration in supine position, and measurement of arterial oxygen saturation during sleep. Correction of nocturnal hypoventilation not only improves cardiac failure symptoms but also decreases the burden on diaphragm during daytime respiration [5].

During REM (Rapid Eye Movement) sleep, the maintenance of ventilation purely depends on diaphragm. Disorders associated with diaphragm weakness due to variable causes (phrenic nerve damage, CMT, COPD) have disturbances in sleep during night time. The diaphragm palsy is associated with reduction in REM sleep. Similarly, in amyotrophic lateral sclerosis patients there is a marked reduction in REM sleep duration and periodic leg movement sequences. There is no marked variation in apnea-hypopnea index except few episodes of obstructive apnea during REM, and central hypopnea during NREM [6].

Another neuropathic disorder that presents with hypoventilation and disordered sleep is multifocal motor neuropathy with conduction block (MMNCB). The patients also complain of early morning headache, daytime sleepiness, frequent snoring, stridor, and episodes of apnea during sleep. Polysomnographic findings include poor sleep efficiency, decreased REM sleep, and very high apnea-hypopnea index. It was possible to demonstrate the most significant cause of patient's daytime sleepiness was sleep-induced hypopnea due to diaphragm weakness in MMNCB. The apnea-hypopnea events recorded in polysomnography study were mainly due to diaphragm weakness due to phrenic nerve involvement but these were also exacerbated by upper airway obstruction. This is one of the reasons why patients with MMNCB don't tolerate CPAP and are minimally responsive to nocturnal bilevel ventilator. Fortunately, MMNCB patients respond well to intravenous immunoglobulin, by reducing conduction block along the phrenic nerve [7].

Sleep apnea itself can be a risk factor for peripheral neuropathy. In hypoxic neuropathy, nerve capillary endothelial cell hyperplasia leads to endoluminal occlusion and thickening of perineurium which can impede the transport of nutrients and oxygen. Several studies indicate that an increased prevalence of polyneuropathy in COPD and OSA patients was due to repetitive hypoxia events during sleep. Patients with OSA have required supramaximal stimulation to obtain sensory and mixed nerve action potentials higher than controls. The reduced amplitude of sensory nerve action potentials in the OSA group indicates axonal damage. Sensory conduction velocity was slower in OSA patients compared to controls, this means, chronic exposure to severe intermittent hypoxia resulting in resistance to ischemic conduction block (RICB) [8]. RICB is likely an adaptation to endoneurial hypoxemia. RICB was disappeared in OSA patients who were treated with prolonged CPAP therapy. The severity of axonal damage in OSA patients was correlated with the percentage of night time with oxygen saturation below 90%. The reversibility of polyneuropathy with prolonged CPAP therapy in OSA patients is still under investigation [9].

Spinocerebellar ataxia (SCA) per se causes peripheral neuropathy and associated with RLS, as we mentioned above that both cause sleep disturbances. SCA patients especially suffer from trouble in falling asleep, nocturnal awakenings, nightmares, and insufficient refreshment after sleep. Long-standing disease, old age, and brain stem involvement in SCA were associated with more frequent sleep problems. Interestingly, CAG repeat length was not associated with sleep issues. Polysomnography reveals reduced sleep stages 3 and 4, REM, and periodic limb movement in sleep. Fifty percent of SCA patients with sleep problems had no history of RLS, this means RLS is not the sole cause for sleep issues in SCA patients [10].

Restless legs syndrome (RLS) can cause severe sleep problems both in initiating and maintaining the sleep. RLS is associated with iron deficiency, diabetes, rheumatoid arthritis, and hypothyroidism. RLS is frequently associated with peripheral neuropathy that leads to sleep disturbances. Neuropathies and radiculopathies have been associated with RLS but their relation is complicated. Neuropathy (both large and small fiber) occurs more frequently in nonfamilial RLS, may involve sensory symptoms, and presents at later ages. While nerve conduction study/EMG is helpful in diagnosing large fiber neuropathy, skin biopsy is useful to identify small fiber neuropathy. There are some case reports that link RLS to CMT, cryoglobulinemic neuropathy, and familial amyloid polyneuropathy [11]. Patients with RLS showed poorer overall quality of sleep, longer sleep latency, shorter sleep duration, less sleep efficiency, and use of more sedatives. RLS patients also have periodic limb movement disorder that further associated with arousal from sleep. Patients with RLS also have periodic limb movements while awake [11]. Treatment with dopaminergic agents has been reported to improve sleep [12].

There is a close relationship between RLS and neuropathy, and polyneuropathy secondary to Lyme's disease had resolution of RLS symptoms as their polyneuropathy improved with antibiotics. These polyneuropathy patients should be asked about motor restlessness; if present, they should be treated with carbidopa/levodopa combination [13].

Here an interesting point is, some authors based on rigorous studies claimed that there is no conclusive evidence that proves an association between diabetes and restless legs syndrome although RLS has been associated with polyneuropathy and diabetes is a common cause of polyneuropathy. Adult type 2 diabetics have higher rates of insomnia, difficulty in sleep onset and maintenance, and also have high ESS over 12. The use of hypnotics was also higher than controls. RLS was common in both groups and it was not statistically significant. They noticed higher prevalence rate of insomnia in diabetics with RLS than without RLS, but it is not statistically significant. RLS occurs in diabetic patients irrespective of medication use, renal insufficiency, and peripheral neuropathy. Neither duration of diabetes nor level of control were significant predictors of RLS [14].

Diabetes is the most common cause of peripheral neuropathy. There is a strong association between painful diabetic neuropathy (DPN) and levels of anxiety, depression, and sleep disturbances [15]. At the same time, impaired sleep dysregulates the glucose metabolism and insulin resistance. Sleep has great modulatory balance in endocrine, metabolic, and autonomic system. Individuals who sleep less than 6 hours per night show alteration in glucose and insulin levels and a decrease in insulin sensitivity [16]. Painful DPN was associated with spectrum of sleep disturbances more than other chronic diseases and PHN. Control of neuropathic pain and of polyuria may be beneficial in reducing sleep disruption in diabetic patients [17].

Adult nonobese diabetics with autonomic neuropathy have obstructive sleep apnea/hypopnea with a frequency of greater than 30% irrespective of their severity of dysautonomia [18].

Non-pharmacological treatment option for DPN includes homeopathy, acupuncture, low intensity laser therapy, and low frequency pulsed magnetic field therapy. Of this, low frequency pulsed magnetic field (PMF) seems beneficial. Some authors claim a positive role of PMF in glycemic control, probable explanation for this was PMF could cause increased insulin secretion and peripheral tissue glucose uptake [19].

Pharmacological treatment with pregabalin has shown efficacy in control of neuropathic pain in patients with peripheral neuropathy. Pregabalin and similar pain modulating medications increase NREM (Non-Rapid Eye Movement) and decrease REM (Rapid Eye Movement) sleep. Onset of improvement in pain and sleep can occur within first week of therapy with these medications. Patients treated with pregabalin reported less tension, anxiety and improvement in mood [20].

Chronic neuropathic pain associated with various comorbidities includes disruption of sleep, anxiety, and depression [21]. Behavioral interventions play a major role in improving sleep in these patients, some of which include relaxation therapy, sleep restriction therapy, and cognitive therapy.

Key Points
1. Half of all cases of apnea in Charcot–Marie–Tooth disease were due to central sleep apnea. Increased sensitivity to carbon dioxide, chemosensitivity and ventilator response to carbon dioxide, reduced $PaCO_2$ in patients with CMT are possible predictive values for central apnea.
2. Sleep apnea itself can be a risk factor for peripheral neuropathy. In hypoxic neuropathy, nerve capillary endothelial cell hyperplasia leads to endoluminal occlusion and thickening of perineurium which can impede the transport of nutrients and oxygen.
3. During REM (Rapid Eye Movement) sleep, the maintenance of ventilation purely depends on diaphragm.
4. In Charcot–Marie–Tooth (CMT) patients, both pharyngeal and laryngeal neuropathy can lead to severe sleep apnea. These neuropathies interfere with functional status of pharyngeal group of muscles and those local reflexes preventing the upper airway collapse during inspiration.
5. In patients with hereditary sensory motor neuropathy who present with symptoms of nocturnal hypoventilation and unexplained cardiac failure, we should suspect the possibility of diaphragmatic weakness.
6. Symptoms of restless legs syndrome occur in diabetic patients irrespective of medication use, renal insufficiency, and peripheral neuropathy. Neither duration of diabetes nor level of control were significant predictors of RLS.
7. Diabetes is the most common cause of peripheral neuropathy. Chronic neuropathic pain associated with various comorbidities includes disruption of sleep, anxiety, and depression.
8. Pregabalin and similar pain modulating medications increase non-rapid eye movement and decrease rapid eye movement sleep.
9. Neuropathy occurs more frequently in nonfamilial RLS, may involve sensory symptoms, and presents at later ages.
10. Patients with multifocal motor neuropathy with conduction block don't tolerate CPAP and are minimally responsive to nocturnal bilevel ventilator. But their sleep disturbances respond well to intravenous immunoglobulin.

References

1. Vernon MK, et al. Reliability, validity, and responsiveness of the daily sleep interference scale among diabetic peripheral neuropathy and postherpetic neuralgia patients. J Pain Symptom Manage. 2008;36(1):54–68.
2. Lévy P, Pépin J-L, Dematteis M. Pharyngeal neuropathy in obstructive sleep apnea: where are we going? Am J Respir Crit Care Med. 2012;185(3):241–3.
3. Dematteis M, et al. Charcot-Marie-Tooth disease and sleep apnoea syndrome: a family study. Lancet. 2001;357(9252):267–72.
4. Dematteis M, Pépin J-L, Lévy P. Central sleep apnoeas in patients with Charcot-Marie-Tooth disease. Lancet. 2001;358(9275):70–1.
5. Hardie R, et al. Diaphragmatic weakness in hereditary motor and sensory neuropathy. J Neurol Neurosurg Psychiatry. 1990;53(4):348–50.

6. Arnulf I, et al. Sleep disorders and diaphragmatic function in patients with amyotrophic lateral sclerosis. Am J Respir Crit Care Med. 2000;161(3):849–56.
7. Kyriakides T, et al. Sleep hypoventilation syndrome and respiratory failure due to multifocal motor neuropathy with conduction block. Muscle Nerve. 2011;43(4):610–4.
8. Mayer P, et al. Peripheral neuropathy in sleep apnea: a tissue marker of the severity of nocturnal desaturation. Am J Respir Crit Care Med. 1999;159(1):213–9.
9. Lüdemann P, et al. Axonal polyneuropathy in obstructive sleep apnoea. J Neurol Neurosurg Psychiatry. 2001;70(5):685–7.
10. Schöls L, et al. Sleep disturbance in spinocerebellar ataxias Is the SCA3 mutation a cause of restless legs syndrome? Neurology. 1998;51(6):1603–7.
11. Kushida CA. Clinical presentation, diagnosis, and quality of life issues in restless legs syndrome. Am J Med. 2007;120(1):S4–S12.
12. Lopes LA, et al. Restless legs syndrome and quality of sleep in type 2 diabetes. Diabetes Care. 2005;28(11):2633–6.
13. Rutkove SB, Matheson JK, Logigian EL. Restless legs syndrome in patients with polyneuropathy. Muscle Nerve. 1996;19(5):670–2.
14. Skomro R, et al. Sleep complaints and restless legs syndrome in adult type 2 diabetics. Sleep Med. 2001;2(5):417–22.
15. Zelman DC, Brandenburg NA, Gore M. Sleep impairment in patients with painful diabetic peripheral neuropathy. Clin J Pain. 2006;22(8):681–5.
16. Trento M, et al. Sleep abnormalities in type 2 diabetes may be associated with glycemic control. Acta Diabetol. 2008;45(4):225–9.
17. Gore M, et al. Pain severity in diabetic peripheral neuropathy is associated with patient functioning, symptom levels of anxiety and depression, and sleep. J Pain Symptom Manage. 2005;30(4):374–85.
18. Bottini P, et al. Sleep-disordered breathing in nonobese diabetic subjects with autonomic neuropathy. Eur Respir J. 2003;22(4):654–60.
19. Wrobel M, et al. Impact of low frequency pulsed magnetic fields on pain intensity, quality of life and sleep disturbances in patients with painful diabetic polyneuropathy. Diabetes Metab. 2008;34(4):349–54.
20. Rosenstock J, et al. Pregabalin for the treatment of painful diabetic peripheral neuropathy: a double-blind, placebo-controlled trial. Pain. 2004;110(3):628–38.
21. Nicholson B, Verma S. Comorbidities in chronic neuropathic pain. Pain Med. 2004;5(s1):S9–S27.

Sleep Issues in Pediatric Neuromuscular Disorders

Raja Boddepalli and Raghav Govindarajan

Introduction

Sleep-related breathing disorders (SRBD) are defined as recurrent, partial, or complete cessation in breathing that disrupts normal sleep and ventilation. These include central apnea, hypoventilation, and the spectrum of obstructive sleep apnea (OSA) attributable to wide array of disorders from simple snoring to complete upper airway closure. Moreover, they are very common in children with neuromuscular disorders (NMD) that can be hereditary or nonhereditary in origin. The prevalence of SRBD in NMD is greater than 40%, i.e., 10 times more than general pediatric population, and suggests the involvement of respiratory muscles. It's quite a challenge in recognition and diagnosis of SRBD, as they are overlooked, unrecognized, or misdiagnosed.

Children with NMD are more prone to hypercapnic hypoventilation and hypoxemia. The adverse pathophysiological changes resulting from NMD compromise ventilatory mechanism and development of hypoxemic conditions that include pulmonary artery hypertension, cor-pulmonale, and neurocognitive dysfunction. The ensuing complications from deranged ventilatory mechanisms in NMD can be further aggravated and fastened with underlying OSAS. The coexistent illnesses contribute for more decreased chemical neuroresponsiveness when compared to children with either disorder alone. Hence, it warrants early recognition and addressing of SRBD and OSAS in children with NMD. If left untreated are likely to contribute greater morbidity, mortality and sleep-related hypoxemic complications when left untreated.

R. Boddepalli, M.D.
Academic Department, Stony Brook University School of Medicine, Stony Brook, NY, USA

R. Govindarajan, M.D., F.A.A.N. (✉)
Department of Neurology, University of Missouri, Columbia, MO, USA
e-mail: govindarajanr@health.missouri.edu

Pediatric Neuromuscular disorders

The most important executive function of sleep is breathing. The diaphragm is the principle muscle for inspiration during wakefulness and sleep.

Respiratory Physiology in Sleep

During stages of REM (Rapid Eye Movement) and NREM (Non-Rapid Eye Movement), there is a decreased sensitivity of respiratory center to chemical and mechanical inputs along with a major decrease in the stimulant effects of cortical inputs. Likewise, upper airway resistance increases during sleep compared to wakefulness, thereby aggravating upper airway occlusion and obstructive sleep apnea syndrome (OSAS) in susceptible individuals. The hypoventilation during sleep is attributable for reduction in oxygen consumption and carbon dioxide production when compared to wakefulness.

In REM sleep, respirations become faster and more irregular. The respiratory frequency persists through hypoxia, hypercapnia, and metabolic alkalosis, suggestive of neurogenic forces superseding chemotactic reflexes during REM sleep. The sensitivity of respiratory muscles to respiratory center outputs is also reduced and more marked in REM sleep. The elemental feature in REM sleep respiratory physiology is that diaphragm assumes all functions of respiration. During REM sleep, there is marked atonia of all muscles (tongue, pharyngeal, laryngeal, intercostal muscles, etc.) of the body except oculomotor muscles and with major incapacitance for any significant function. In addition, there appears to be supraspinal inhibition of γ-motor neurons (and to a lesser extent α-motor neurons) and presynaptic inhibition of afferent terminals from muscle spindles. The diaphragm, being driven almost entirely by α-motor neurons and with far fewer spindles than intercostal muscles, has little tonic (postural) activity and therefore escapes reduction of this drive during REM sleep. This helps to explain the increase in abdominal contribution to breathing in REM sleep.

In NREM, sensitivity of diaphragm to respiratory center output is more when compared to accessory muscles and along with notable breathing that is regular both in amplitude and frequency.

In sleep, ventilatory drive in response to hypoxia and hypercapnia is also reduced. In NREM, there is a decrease in minute ventilation, largely due to a rise in end-tidal carbon dioxide tension ($PETCO_2$).

Neuromuscular disorders are broad distinct diseases that involve nerves, muscles, or their connections. Likewise, these disorders may share common features of reduced diaphragmatic strength, weakness of upper airway dilators, or cardiomyopathy that contributes to the development of SRBD. The diaphragmatic weakness in children with NMD is primarily responsible and detrimental for ventilatory compromise. It is markedly evident in REM sleep, at a time when diaphragm is the only effective respiratory pump. NMD patients with diaphragmatic weakness rely on intercostal and accessory respiratory muscles to breathe; when these muscles become atonic in REM sleep, they are prone to hypoventilation. Thus, predisposing children with NMD to hypercapnic hypoventilation and first evidenced during REM sleep. Hence, two different types of sleep-associated nocturnal respiratory disorders are seen in children with neuromuscular weakness:

1. Obstructive sleep Apnea
2. Nocturnal hypoventilation

Sleep-related central hypoventilation is the primary pattern of SRBD in children with Duchenne Muscular Dystrophy (DMD), Spinal Muscular Atrophy (SMA), congenital myotonic dystrophy, limb-girdle muscular dystrophies, and childhood-onset maltase acid deficiency (see Table 7.2). Likewise, children with myotonic dystrophy, congenital muscular dystrophy, congenital non-progressive myopathies, spinal muscular atrophy, and myasthenia gravis exhibit sleep-related chronic obstructive hypoventilation because of a combination pharyngeal muscle weakness, predisposing to upper airway collapse, chest and abdominal wall weakness.

Sleep-Related Clinical Manifestations in NMD

SRBD are common in children with NMD, occur irrespective to the pathogenesis of each of these disorders, and manifest especially during REM sleep. These symptoms can be detected even when muscle weakness is still mild and even with no evidence of diurnal respiratory dysfunction. Labanowski et al., in a prospective study of 60 neuromuscular patients demonstrated disturbed sleep, snoring and restless legs in a majority of them (both adult and pediatric).

The children present with diverse symptoms and are isolated which include nocturnal restlessness, frequent unexplained awakenings and with awakenings gasping for air, snoring of variable loudness along with lapses in respiratory activity, difficulty waking up in morning and with prolonged sleep inertia. During daytime, there is excessive somnolence, fatigue, and inappropriate napping that lead to failure to thrive in the infant and poor school grades in the child. In addition, changes in mood, attention deficit, and learning difficulties are also observed. In severe cases, patients exhibit nocturnal cyanosis, intractable insomnia, morning lethargy, early morning headaches, nausea, vomiting, and hypoxia-induced nocturnal seizures. Polycythemia, hypertension, and signs of heart failure can also be seen. Sitting positions at night, nocturnal cyanosis, severe morning lethargy, headaches, and vomiting indicate advanced neuromuscular impediment to ventilation in sleep.

Likewise, sleep-related clinical symptoms result from hypoventilation and become more prominent and severe with progression of disease. Children with sleep-related ventilatory deficits exhibit continuous nocturnal hypoxemia or triggering episodes of oxygen desaturation that can precipitate restlessness, arousals, and sleep fragmentation.

Nevertheless, symptoms are poorly predictive of SRBD in children with NMD. It is even more difficult in children with low intellectual functioning. They can be minimal despite significant apneas and severe nocturnal oxygen desaturations. Likewise, some report symptoms suggesting nocturnal hypoventilation, but these may be misinterpreted as part of the progressive deterioration of the underlying neuromuscular disorder.

Diagnostic and Clinical Evaluation of SRBD

Respiratory insufficiency in children with NMD is an early indicator for a progressive disease. Moreover, impairment of respiratory muscles occurs in various NMD and in some they are progressive to non-ambulatory stage. According to the International Classification of Sleep Disorders (ICSD)-3 (2014), neurological disorders for causation of SRBD are diagnosed distinctly and are included in clinical division of sleep-related breathing disorders and cited under sleep-related hypoventilation due to a medical disorder (see Table 7.1). Here the "medical disorder" is comprehensive and includes lung parenchymal or airway disease, pulmonary vascular pathology, chest wall disorder, neurologic disorder such as neuromuscular disorders (disorders of brain, spinal cord, or phrenic nerve), and myopathies. The current ICSD-3 criteria for sleep-related hypoventilation in pediatric age group is in synonymous with hypoventilation, as defined in AASM scoring manual: Hypoventilation is scored when the arterial PCO_2 (or surrogate) is >50 mmHg for >25% of total sleep time. The surrogates of arterial PCo_2 are end-tidal PCO_2 or transcutaneous PCO_2 (diagnostic study) or transcutaneous PCO_2 (titration study).

Clinical History

A focused clinical history and certain components of physical examination on background of ongoing NMD can aid in evaluating sleep-related breathing disorders.

The patient should be evaluated for craniofacial abnormalities such as micrognathia, dental malocclusion, high arched palate, etc., as they are commonly observed in NMD and compromise oropharyngeal lumen. Likewise, anatomical changes in the oropharyngeal region including tonsillar hypertrophy and macroglossia (sometimes seen in hypothyroidism or acromegaly) may also be present in

Table 7.1 ICSD-3 criteria: Sleep-related hypoventilation due to a medical disorder

1. Sleep-related hypoventilation is present
2. A lung parenchymal or airway disease, pulmonary vascular pathology, chest wall disorder, neurologic disorder, or muscular weakness is believed to be the primary cause of hypoventilation
3. Hypoventilation is not primarily due to obesity hypoventilation syndrome, medication use or a known congenital central alveolar hypoventilation syndrome

patients with neuromuscular disease. Kyphoscoliosis that is commonly observed in patients with NMD inhibits chest and abdominal movement, as postural alteration of the spine in conjunction with NMD-related weakness causes dysfunction of diaphragm and intercostal muscles, thereby translating into a less-efficient respiratory mechanism.

The presence of weak cough reflexes, obesity, restrictive pulmonary disease, medication effects, and malnutrition should be ruled out as these exacerbate SRBD in children with NMD.

Predictors for SRBD in Children with NMD

The principal effect with impairment of respiratory muscles in NMD is compromise of ventilatory mechanisms. Serial monitoring of pulmonary functioning tests, in children with NMD, once they are capable to participate in testing (>5 years) may aid in predicting which NMD patients are more likely to have sleep-related hypoventilation. Likewise, it assists in affirming rather than concluding SRBD merely basing on symptoms. Sleep-related central hypoventilation can likely be present in a child with NMD when inspiratory vital capacity falls below 40% of predicted or 60% of predicted in obese children, concomitant lung disease or during lung infection and a daytime $paCO_2$ level of >40 mmHg. Mellies et al. have found that IVC <40% of predicted had a 96% sensitivity and 88% specificity and daytime $paCO_2$ level >40 mmHg had a 92% sensitivity and 72% specificity in predicting sleep-related hypoventilation in children with NMD.

Assessment of SRBD

There are various clinically available tests to assess SRBD and with varying utility. The appropriate test that can be administered in an ideal clinical setting remains inconclusive. The gold standard method to document hypoventilation is by determining arterial partial pressure of carbon dioxide ($PaCO_2$) through processing of an arterial blood sample. However, limited by difficulty of drawing blood in sleep, 2007 AASM scoring manual states finding an elevated $PaCO_2$ obtained immediately after waking would provide evidence of hypoventilation during sleep. Nonetheless the elusiveness of recording sleeping $PaCO_2$, the ability to draw or process an arterial blood gas sample is rarely available in sleep centers.

Diurnal Tests

The diurnal clinical symptoms, evaluation and assessment tools yield some clues in early recognition of SRBD in children with NMD. These can be contributory as well as can be non-contributory in diagnosing SRBD.

The diurnal symptoms including morning headaches, lethargy, and daytime sleepiness are evident with either rapid or slower progression of NMD. The majority of diurnal symptoms in Labanowski et al. study of 60 adult and pediatric patients with various NMD were fatigue (83%), exertional dyspnea (78%), daytime sleepiness (63%), and morning headaches (45%). In addition, mean Epworth Sleepiness Scale score (ESS) in this study population was 7.5. Despite high reporting of SRBD in the study, symptoms along with ESS were not predictive of its occurrence.

Pediatric sleep-related questionnaires that are used to investigate or evaluate sleep issues in children remain inconclusive in majority cases including evaluation of OSA.

At the same time, it is challenging for parents in administering these questionnaires for:

1. Limited understanding on hypoventilation based on elusive symptomatology and signs of SRBD in a progressive NMD.
2. The limitation in predicting and assessing severity of SRBD based on these manifestations is always uncertain.

Pulmonary function tests are valuable in investigating and monitoring of response to treatment in patients with sleep-related respiratory problems. Hukins and Hillman in their prospective study of 19 patients with DMD have established forced expiratory volume in 1 s (FEV_1) < 40% and 20% than predicted was sensitive for presence of SRBD and daytime retention of Co_2, respectively.

Diurnal Polysomnography (PSG)

Polysomnography or formal sleep study remains the gold-standard test in diagnosing SRBD. Several studies have investigated the utility and reliability of daytime nap polysomnography (DPSG) versus nocturnal polysomnography (NPSG) in diagnosing SRBD. They have found DPSG is not as sensitive as NPSG in identifying SRBD. On the other hand, they tend to underestimate the severity of SRBD when compared to NPSG.

The measurement of PCo_2 reflects the effectiveness of alveolar ventilation and its measurement by sampling either capillary or arterial blood can estimate hypoventilation. The daytime capillary or arterial blood PCo_2 > 45 arguably suggest for nocturnal hypoventilation and reasoning for an early intervention and evaluation.

Nocturnal Tests

Polysomnography (PSG)

A comprehensive overnight PSG is the gold-standard test for assessing SRBD in children with NMD. The study involves a continuous non-invasive monitoring and assessments are ascertained based on observational recordings from video, electroencephalogram (EEG), electromyogram (EMG), oxygen saturation and carbon dioxide level as well as chest and abdominal wall movements. The cohesive assessment helps in evaluation of cardiorespiratory compromise in association with sleep and altered sleep architecture (Reduced sleep time + Sleep efficiency), apart from differentiating seizures, periodic limb movements, and other parasomnias.

Katz et al. in their prospective study demonstrated that a series of single night PSG, was a valid measure and was without significant night to night variations in respiratory parameters. In addition, the study establishes clinical utility and predictability of PSG as a diagnostic tool in SRBD. The practice parameters from American Academy of sleep medicine indicate PSG in patients with neuromuscular disorders, manifesting sleep-related clinical symptoms with unequivocal and no plausible clinical explanation. The overnight PSG should be performed:

1. As early as possible in all neuromuscular patients for a baseline recording of respiratory parameters and repeated depending on course of the neuromuscular disease.
2. Regularly after initiation of treatment for assessment of treatment efficacy.

However, the test is limited for needing specialist centers and along with long wait times in scheduling and reimbursements. Likewise, it is expensive, labor intensive and might be disruptive for families. Moreover, there is a likely interference from monitoring with sleep, limiting REM during which SRBD manifests.

Overnight Oximetry

It is a non-invasive test and more widely available as it can be performed in a patient's home. Brouillette et al. has suggested a positive nocturnal oximetry trend graph has at least a 97% positive predictive value in child suspected of having OSA. Walsh et al. has demonstrated the reduction in requirement of formal PSG by 70% with use of domiciliary overnight oximetry.

The events of repetitive clusters of "saw tooth" desaturation may occur in children with OSA during REM sleep and prolonged periods of desaturation are observed with hypoventilation. The test has its own limitations: (1) It fails to interpret severity of SRBD as it hastens for early initiation of medical management. (2) Normal pulse oximetry cannot rule out the presence of SRBD as respiratory events attributed to arousals rather from desaturations are not detected. (3) The technical problems like motion artifact and as well as long built-in averaging time of the device can result either in overestimation or underestimation of respiratory events.

The search for simpler and other sophisticated ambulatory testing in assessment of SRBD has been ongoing. Home-made audio and video recordings lack sensitivity and specificity to diagnose SRBD. Kirk et al. study has demonstrated using capnography alone in diagnosing SRBD was not clear. The addition of capnography to oximetry, probably as an adjunct tool in diagnosing SRBD has been suggested.

However, the proposed role of capnography as an adjunct to oximetry in diagnosing SRBD warrants more studies.

Management of SRBD

Treatment

Over the years, advances in diagnosis and supportive care as such in ventilatory support or rehabilitative therapies have substantially improved functional status and survival in NMD children with SRBD.

The management of respiratory insufficiency during sleep is quite a challenge for: (1) It requires appropriate therapeutic intervention directed in augmenting the underlying disorder. (2) The applicable pharmacological therapies and time in initiation of either non-invasive or invasive ventilation is unclear.

There are different patterns of SRBD like apnea, obstructive apneas, hypopneas, central apneas, and frank central hypoventilation in children with NMD. For an optimal treatment, it is highly suggested for differentiating various apneas at diagnostic workup. The most common form of sleep-disordered breathing is hypoventilation and as such oxygen therapy alone is not only mostly ineffective, but may even be harmful, worsening the severity of CO_2 retention. Nowadays, non-invasive ventilation (NIV) has become a standard of treatment for an effective improvement in blood gases and reducing need for invasive ventilation. Ward et al. in their randomized control trial demonstrated beneficial effects of long-term non-invasive ventilation in patients with nocturnal hypoventilation and daytime normocapnia. Likewise, Piper and Sullivan study has demonstrated the importance of long-term nocturnal NIV in reducing severity of nocturnal hypoventilation.

The initial approach to treat SRBD in children with NMD is application of non-invasive positive pressure ventilation (NIPPV) during sleep. It has been effective in treatment of SRBD and hypoventilation in Duchenne muscular dystrophy (DMD) and various NMD. It is usually recommended:

1. Respiratory insufficiency unravels underlying NMD.
2. Chronic daytime respiratory failure.
3. Sleep-related hypoventilation is believed to be resulting from muscular weakness or NMD.

Non-invasive Positive Pressure Ventilation (NIPPV)

NIPPV is delivery of mechanical ventilation by augmenting alveolar ventilation and creating a transpulmonary pressure gradient without need for an indwelling artificial airway. The goals of NIPPV are firstly to improve gas exchanges by improving tidal volumes (VT) and secondly to decrease work of respiratory muscle. Likewise, it can contribute in resetting chemosensitivity of respiratory center. There is no clear consensus in recommending long-term mechanical ventilation in cases of severe progressive neuromuscular disorders, as pros and cons of such are debatable. Even in such patients, NIPPV offers a meaningful hope of modality in maintaining reasonable alveolar ventilation without tracheostomy. Hence, NIPPV is attributable for improved quality of sleep, daytime sleepiness, quality of life, with an overall improvement in respiratory distress index and increasing longevity. The modes of delivery of NIPPV are bi-level positive airway pressure ventilation (BiPAP), volume-cycled ventilation, and continuous positive airway pressure (CPAP).

BiPAP is not as efficacious as volume-cycled ventilation when given through mask. Furthermore, BiPAP devices generate maximum inspiratory pressure of 30 cm H_2O resulting in low delivery of VT when compared to volume-cycled ventilation. Conversely, BiPAP ventilatory support is less complicated to initiate and less costly. BiPAP or volume-cycled ventilation can be considered in clinical situations where hypoxemia completely or in part results from hypoventilation. The role of CPAP as a first-line treatment in children with NMD warrants more studies. However, CPAP may be beneficial in children with suspected obstructive sleep apnea in absence of hypoventilation. For most NMD and predominantly children with DMD, CPAP remains ineffective as thoracoabdominal impairment is principal cause for sleep-related respiratory disturbances.

The optimal positive pressures required to reduce obstructive sleep apneas or hypopneas and stabilize ventilation should be determined either in sleep laboratory or by careful bedside monitoring and observation. After application of NIPPV, it is essential for a close bedside assessment of its effectiveness by the respiratory care team, including the physician. Furthermore, children treated with NIPPV must be observed by qualified professional staff using cardiac and respiratory monitors, pulse oximetry, and blood gases as and when necessary.

The complications commonly encountered with delivery of NIPPV include injury to face secondary to mask, eye irritation, conjunctivitis, skin necrosis/ulceration, gastric distension, and emesis into facial mask. The eye irritation can be minimized with use of appropriate fitting equipment and clear occlusive dressing. Similarly, skin necrosis/ulceration can be minimized either with use of a properly fitting mask or by use of a patch or skin dressing applied to skin pressure point. The other uncommon serious complications that need to be vigilant are for aspiration and pneumothorax.

Invasive Mechanical Ventilation

The increased respiratory exertion resulting either from progression of NMD as such or secondary to superimposed infections furthers for more stabilization of ventilation and may even necessitate for invasive ventilation. The consensus on indication for invasive ventilation is subjective. Conversely, it is critical as part of supportive care in children with advanced NMD and compromised respiratory status. The common indications for need of mechanical ventilation: (1) Upper airway compromise resulting from weakness of facial, oropharyngeal, and laryngeal muscles impedes secretion clearance and swallowing. Consequently, placing the patient at risk for aspiration and causing mechanical obstruction of the upper airway. (2) The weakness of inspiratory muscles compromising expansion of lung by causing microatelectasis, ventilation/perfusion mismatch and with resultant hypoxemia. Likewise, weakness of expiratory muscles causes ineffective cough and secretion clearance and with increased risk for aspiration and pneumonia. (3) The acute complications of illnesses like pneumonia or pulmonary embolism may worsen the already compromised respiratory system.

It is essential to be watchful for complications as they can occur at any period of invasive mechanical ventilation and some are life threatening. A few which include: (1) ventilator-induced lung injury (2) Barotrauma and volutrauma, and (3) Ventilator-Associated Pneumonia (VAP).

However, it is well established that NIV is much superior to invasive mechanical ventilation in patients with NMD needing long-term ventilatory support. NIV takes precedence for (1) Very economical and with ease of administration. (2) Less burden on caregivers. (3) Greater portability (4) Potential reduction and elimination of airway complications (5) Reduced need for hospitalization.

Interfaces

The modality of NIPPV involves delivery of pressurized gas to lungs through a mask or mouthpiece that is affixed to the nose, mouth, or both. The clinically relevant issue is to select an appropriate interface with due consideration for patient comfort and minimal leakage. Moreover, selection of a larger nasal mask in view of patient comfort has adverse clinical effects:

1. The need for extreme pressures to secure mask would result in dermal abrasion around margins of mask.
2. The larger masks in children enclosing both oral and nasal passages with intent to minimize leaks contribute for an increased risk for aspiration pneumonia, gastric distension with air, feeding difficulties, and worsening of gastro-esophageal reflux.

In children needing long-term NIPPV, nasal mask interface would be an ideal choice either to maintain or to regulate required peak inspiratory pressures. The nasal-oral masks can be used safely in children provided there is reasonable level of monitoring. In acute settings, nasal-oral mask is superior to nasal masks in reducing oral leaks. The initial experiences with newly available interfaces, providing NIPPV in children like helmet device, nasal pillows or plugs and modified wide-bore soft nasal tubing systems are promising. However, experiences with these devices are preliminary, warranting more studies.

Home Mechanical Ventilation

The institution of home mechanical ventilation (HMV) has shown to prolong and improve quality of life in children with NMD. The number of children on home mechanical ventilation is reported to be increasing and has been well accepted as a standard treatment in children with chronic respiratory failure. HMV is favorable in children developing progressive respiratory failure or intractable failure to wean mechanical ventilation. Besides, HMV can also be helpful in children with increased respiratory load from airway or lung pathologies, ventilatory muscle weakness, and failure of neurologic control of ventilation. However, lack of studies limits consensus on guidelines of institution of HMV.

Special Disorders

Duchenne Muscular Dystrophy (DMD)

DMD is X-linked form of muscular dystrophy characterized by a defect in gene that affects synthesis of dystrophin protein. The clinical symptoms manifest between 3 and 4 years of age and with gradual deterioration in muscle function. With the gradual progression, children become less ambulant and wheel chair dependent before their adolescence. However, steroids have been effective in prolonging ambulation and improving respiratory muscle strength and clinical outcome. Likewise, ambulation, extent, and rate of progression of weakness in respiratory muscles causing respiratory insufficiency, daytime and nocturnal gas exchange impairment can aid in assessing clinical outcome and longevity.

The SRBD associated with DMD is more common in REM sleep and is demonstrated with significant drop in minute ventilation when compared to NREM. The impaired ventilator drive is a possible mechanism in these patients. There is a bimodal presentation of SRBD, with manifestation of OSA in first decade and hypoventilation more commonly at the beginning of the second decade. Their initial presentation is very subtle to notice and include continuing increasing numbers of nocturnal awakenings, daytime somnolence, fatigue, and morning headaches. In addition, these patients are at more risk of developing upper airway obstruction.

The aforesaid complaints when reported by patients should especially be drawn attention for a thorough evaluation by a physician. However, there are no clear guidelines for timing of polysomnography in patients with DMD. As such one study has correlated sleep hypoventilation with an awake $PaCo_2$ of >45 mmHg and a base excess >4 mmol/L. In another study, sleep study alone in home has demonstrated SRBD in children with SRBD.

The treatment of SRBD in Duchenne's muscular dystrophy with non invasive ventilation.

Spinal Muscular Atrophy (SMA)

SMA is a disorder that affects motor neurons of spinal cord and brain stem, thereby causing weakness of muscle and atrophy. The types of SMA in children are as listed in Table 7.2. It is the second most common NMD in children with an incidence of 8 per 100,000 live births.

SRBD is common in all forms of SMA and along with alterations in sleep architecture. The children presenting with sleep problems, daytime somnolence, morning headaches, and attention deficit during daytime necessitates for a thorough evaluation. The other most common and serious complication of SMA that can cause insidious onset of sleep hypoventilation is restrictive lung disease.

Table 7.2 Major neuromuscular disorders in children and along with type of SRBD

Neuromuscular disease	Mode of inheritance	Gene location	Type of SRBD
1. Duchenne muscular dystrophy (DMD)	XLR	Xp21	Hypoventilation, OSA
2. Becker muscular dystrophy	XLR	Xp21	Hypoventilation, OSA
3. Limb-girdle muscular dystrophy (LGMD)			
(a) LGMD1A	AD	5q22-q34	Hypoventilation
(b) LGMD2B	AR	2p13-2p16	
(c) LGMD2C	AR	13q12	
(d) LGMD2A	AR	15q15.1	
(e) LGMD2D	AR	17q12-q21.33	
4. Facioscapulohumeral muscular dystrophy			Hypoventilation, OSA
5. Emery-Dreifuss	AD	4q35 deletion	Hypoventilation
6. Congenital muscular dystrophies	XLR	Xq28,	OSA, hypoventilation
7. Myotonic dystrophy	AR	6q, 9q31-q33, unknown.	CA, OSA, hypoventilation
8. Spinal muscular atrophy	AD	19q13.2	
(a) Type I (Werdnig–Hoffman disease)	AR	5q11-5q13.	OSA, hypoventilation
(b) Type II (intermediate severity)	AR		
(c) Type III (Kugelberg–Welander disease)	AD, AR.		
9. Congenital Myasthenic syndrome	Unknown		Hypoventilation
10. Congenital myopathies	Unknown		OSA, hypoventilation

AD autosomal dominant, *AR* autosomal recessive, *XLR* X-linked recessive, *CA* central apnea, *OSA* obstructive sleep apnea

Mellies et al. in their study have demonstrated that NIV was an effective long-term treatment of hypoventilation during sleep and respiratory failure. Non-invasive ventilation during sleep eliminates SDB and normalizes sleep architecture in these children. Conversely, ideal settings for commencing NIV have not been clearly established. In some children, the decision to start NIV in prolonging survival may pose ethical conundrum. Even in such cases where NIV cannot prolong survival, it may aid in alleviating symptoms and allowing child to be cared at home.

Limb-Girdle Muscular Dystrophy (LGMD)

LGMD is a broad term for group of disorders causing weakness and wasting of girdle musculature. They are highly heterogeneous both clinically and genetically. The various types of LGMD are as listed in Table 7.2. The various forms of LGMD have childhood onset and may have severe progression resembling DMD. The type of SRBD noted in these children is similar to children with DMD.

Myotonic Dystrophy (MD)

Myotonic dystrophy is most common autosomal dominant disorder affecting children and adults. It is multi-organ disease affecting the muscles, brain, heart, gastrointestinal tract, lens, and reproductive organs. The incidence is 1:8000 births. SRBD has been reported up to 34% of patients with MD.

The children manifest extreme daytime somnolence, sleep fragmentation and these may even present before weakening of respiratory muscles. Similarly, learning disabilities may be noted in childhood-onset myotonic dystrophy type-1 disorder. In addition to respiratory-related arousals, it has been found that about a 1/3 of children has evidence of periodic limb movement during sleep, leading to sleep fragmentation.

Conclusion

The NMD are heterogeneous and have detrimental effects on respiratory function and sleep. Besides, progressive muscle weakness compromises function of upper respiratory system, cough, and clearance of secretions. Nonetheless, initial manifestations of sleep-related symptoms resulting from NMD are very subtle. The severity of SRBD-related symptoms depends on the distribution, rate of progression, and form of neuromuscular defects. Any alarming SRBD-related manifestations warrant for regular assessment of respiratory function during wakefulness and sleep in these patients. As such hypoxemia and hypoventilation are common during sleep; the timely initiation of clinical interventions may improve the quality of life and diminish the high morbidity and mortality associated with NMD.

Key Points
1. Sleep-related breathing disorder in children can present with diverse symptoms and are isolated which include nocturnal restlessness, frequent unexplained awakenings and with awakenings gasping for air, snoring with variable loudness along with lapses in respiratory activity, difficulty waking up in morning and with prolonged sleep inertia.
2. Children with sleep-related ventilatory deficits exhibit continuous nocturnal hypoxemia or triggering episodes of oxygen desaturation that can precipitate restlessness, arousals, and sleep fragmentation.
3. Positive oximetry testing has a high positive predictive value in identifying sleep apnea in children. The oximetry graph shows a typical saw tooth pattern.
4. Sleep-related breathing disorder is common in all forms of spinal muscular atrophy along with alterations in sleep architecture.
5. The sleep-related breathing disorder associated with Duchenne muscular dystrophy is more common in REM sleep and is demonstrated with significant drop in minute ventilation when compared to NREM.
6. In children needing long-term NIPPV, nasal mask interface would be an ideal choice either to maintain or to regulate required peak inspiratory pressures.

Suggested Reading

Aboussouan LS. Sleep-disordered breathing in neuromuscular disease. Am J Respir Crit Care Med. 2015;191(9):979–89.

Alves RSC, Resende MBD, Skomro RP, Souza FJFB, Reed UC. Sleep and neuromuscular disorders in children. Sleep Med Rev. 2009;13(2):133–48.

American Thoracic Society. Standards and indications for cardiopulmonary sleep studies in children. Am J Respir Crit Care Med. 1996;153(2):866–78.

Arens R, Muzumdar H. Sleep, sleep disordered breathing, and nocturnal hypoventilation in children with neuromuscular diseases. Pediatr Respir Rev. 2010;11(1):24–30.

Aurora RN, Zak RS, Karippot A, et al. Practice parameters for the respiratory indications for polysomnography in children. Sleep. 2011;34(3):379–88.

Brouillette RT, Morielli A, Leimanis A, et al. Nocturnal pulse oximetry as an abbreviated testing modality for pediatric obstructive sleep apnea. Pediatrics. 2000;105:405–12.

Buu MC. Respiratory complications, management and treatments for neuromuscular disease in children. Curr Opin Pediatr. 2017;29(3):326–33.

Castro-Codesal ML, Dehaan K, Featherstone R, Bedi PK, Martinez Carrasco C, Katz SL, Chan EY, Bendiak GN, Almeida FR, Olmstead DL, Young R, Woolf V, Waters KA, Sullivan C, Hartling L, MacLean JE. Long-term non-invasive ventilation therapies in children: a scoping review. Sleep Med Rev. 2017;37:148–58.

Chervin RD, Hedger K, Dillon JE, Pituch KJ. Pediatric sleep questionnaire (PSQ): validity and reliability of scales for sleep-disordered breathing, snoring, sleepiness, and behavioral problems. Sleep Med. 2000;1(1):21–32.

Clinical indications for noninvasive positive pressure ventilation in chronic respiratory failure due to restrictive lung disease, COPD, and nocturnal hypoventilation: a consensus conference report. Chest. 1999; 116(2):521–34.

Dorris L, et al. Sleep problems in children with neurological disorders. Dev Neurorehabil. 2008;11(2):95–114.

Frates RC, Splaingard ML, Smith EO, Harrison GM. Outcome of home mechanical ventilation in children. J Pediatr. 1985;106(5):850–6.

Gonzalez Cortés R, Bustinza Arriortua A, Pons Ódena M, García Teresa MA, Cols Roig M, Gaboli M, et al. Domiciliary mechanical ventilation in children: a Spanish multicenter study. An Pediatr. 2013;78(4):227e33.

Guilleminault C, Philip P, Robinson A. Sleep and neuromuscular disease: bilevel positive airway pressure by nasal mask as a treatment for sleep disordered breathing in patients with neuromuscular disease. J Neurol Neurosurg Psychiatry. 1998;65(2):225–32.

Ho G, Widger J, Cardamone M, Farrar MA. Quality of life and excessive daytime sleepiness in children and adolescents with myotonic dystrophy type 1. Sleep Med. 2017;32:92–6.

Hukins CA, Hillman DR. Daytime predictors of sleep hypoventilation in Duchenne muscular dystrophy. Am J Respir Crit Care Med. 2000;161:166–70.

ICSD-2. The international classification of sleep disorders, diagnostic and coding manual. 2nd ed. Westchester, IL: AASM; 2005. p. 74e6. [EUA. P. Hauri, Task Force Chair]

Katz SL. Assessment of sleep-disordered breathing in pediatric neuromuscular diseases. Pediatrics. 2009;123(Suppl4):S222–5.

Katz ES, Greene MG, Carson KA, Galster P, Loughlin GM, Carroll J, et al. Night-to-night variability of polysomnography in children with suspected obstructive sleep apnea. J Pediatr. 2002;140(5):589–94.

Katz S, Selvadurai H, Keilty K, Mitchell M, MacLusky I. Outcome of non-invasive positive pressure ventilation in paediatric neuromuscular disease. Arch Dis Child. 2004;89(2):121–4.

Kirk VG, Flemons WW, Adams C, Rimmer KP, Montgomery MD. Sleep-disordered breathing in duchenne muscular dystrophy: a preliminary study of the role of portable monitoring. Pediatr Pulmonol. 2000;29:135–40.

Labanowski M, Schmidt-Nowara W, Guilleminault C. Sleep and neuromuscular disease: frequency of sleep-disordered breathing in a neuromuscular disease clinic population. Neurology. 1996;47(5):1173–80.

Marcus CL. Sleep-disordered breathing in children. Am J Respir Crit Care Med. 2001;164(1):16–30.

Mellies U, Ragette R, Schwake C, Boehm H, Voit T, Teschler H. Daytime predictors of sleep disordered breathing in children and adolescents with neuromuscular disorders. Neuromuscul Disord. 2003;13:123e8.

Mellies U, Dohna-Schwake C, Stehling F, Voit T. Sleep disordered breathing in spinal muscular atrophy. Neuromuscul Disord. 2004;14(12):797–803.

Messner AH, Pelayo R. Pediatric sleep-related breathing disorders. Am J Otolaryngol. 2000;21(2):98–107. Review

Mindell JA, Owens JA. A clinical guide to pediatric sleep: diagnosis and management of sleep problems. Philadelphia: Lippincott Williams & Wilkins; 2015.

Panitch HB. Respiratory issues in the management of children with neuromuscular disease. Respir Care. 2006;51(8):885e93.

Piper AJ, Sullivan CE. Effects of long-term nocturnal nasal ventilation on spontaneous breathing during sleep in neuromuscular and chest wall disorders. Eur Respir J. 1996;9(7):1515–22.

Practice parameters for the indications for polysomnography and related Procedures. Polysomnography Task Force, American Sleep Disorders Association Standards of Practice Committee. Sleep. 1997;20(6):406–22. (No authors Listed).

Ragette R, Mellies U, Schwake C, Voit T, Teschler H. Patterns and predictors of sleep disordered breathing in primary myopathies. Thorax. 2002;57(8):724e8.

Suresh S, Wales P, Dakin C, Harris MA, Cooper DG. Sleep-related breathing disorder in Duchenne muscular dystrophy: disease spectrum in the paediatric population. J Paediatr Child Health. 2005;41:500e3.

Teague WG. Non-invasive positive pressure ventilation: current status in paediatric patients. Paediatr Respir Rev. 2005;6(1):52–60.
Thorpy MJ. Classification of sleep disorders. Neurotherapeutics. 2012;9(4):687–701.
Wise MS, Nichols CD, et al. Executive summary of respiratory indications for polysomnography in children: an evidence-based review. Sleep. 2011;34(3):389–398AW.
Young HK, Lowe A, Fitzgerald DA, Seton C, Waters KA, Kenny E, Hynan LS, Iannaccone ST, North KN, Ryan MM. Outcome of noninvasive ventilation in children with neuromuscular disease. Neurology. 2007;68(3):198–201.

Basics and Practical Aspects of Non-invasive Mechanical Ventilation

8

Joe Devasahayam, Troy Whitacre, and Tony Oliver

Introduction

Non-invasive ventilation (NIV) is defined as the provision of respiratory support to patients with respiratory failure without invasive means such as with an endotracheal or tracheostomy tube. This lifesaving therapy is used commonly across the healthcare system and since its introduction, has evolved to include a plethora of modes and functionalities. Utilized extensively since the 1980s, NIV has undergone tremendous improvements and is being used in patients with a variety of medical conditions including various neurological disorders that frequently lead to respiratory failure. Despite limitations and the need for careful patient selection, NIV has proven physiological benefits. This includes improved gas exchange and avoids many of the risks associated with invasive mechanical ventilation. Risks include but are not limited to vocal cord injury and ventilator-associated pneumonias—both of which are lessened with NIV. Breaks from NIV allow the possibility for speech and oral intake, thus preserving and extending functionality and quality. In this chapter, we will analyze the general principles and history of mechanical ventilation, the basics of NIV, clinical application, and potential complications and contraindications.

J. Devasahayam, M.D. (✉)
University of Missouri, Columbia, MO, USA

T. Whitacre, R.R.T.
Respiratory Therapy Services, University of Missouri Hospital and Clinics, Columbia, MO, USA
e-mail: whitacret@health.missouri.edu

T. Oliver, M.D.
Sanford Medical Center, University of South Dakota, 1301 S Cliff Ave, Suite 601, Sioux Falls, SD 57105, USA
e-mail: tonyiynas@yahoo.com

© Springer International Publishing AG, part of Springer Nature 2018
R. Govindarajan, P. C. Bollu (eds.), *Sleep Issues in Neuromuscular Disorders*, https://doi.org/10.1007/978-3-319-73068-4_8

History of Artificial Ventilation

Although rudimentary means of artificial ventilation date back as early as the seventeenth century [1], primitive negative pressure ventilators were available in the mid-nineteenth century [2]. The mechanics of these different models were all the same—encasing the chest and passively expanding the thoracic cavity during inspiration by creating negative pressure around the chest wall. Negative pressure ventilators commonly referred to as "iron lungs" evolved, and were used extensively during the mid-twentieth century polio epidemic [3]. Powered by electric motors and air pumps, these ventilators have all but disappeared from the modern clinical setting. Interestingly, there are reports from 2014 that up to ten patients still live in an iron lung [4]. One reason these machines fell out of favor was that caregivers had no access to the patients' torso while they were being actively ventilated. This made routine nursing care impossible. To combat these difficulties, more advanced versions like the "respirator room" and "pneumatic chambers" were designed. In the course of time, negative pressure ventilators were replaced by positive pressure valves that applied pressure to the respiratory system through a tracheostomy tube. Subsequently, cuffed oral as well as nasal endotracheal tubes were developed to avoid the surgical intubation of the trachea. This prevented many of the complications associated with tracheostomies. Complications of invasive methods include vocal cord trauma, bleeding, infection, tracheal injury, stenosis, stricture, and even perforation. However, the inability to speak and increased sedation requirement often associated with invasive ventilation can be mitigated with the application of non-invasive ventilation.

Non-invasive ventilators deliver positive pressure through a snug fitting mask, nasal pillows, or a variety of other interfaces rather than an artificial tube. Initially used to treat obstructive sleep apnea, early machines had very limited setting options. But success with non-invasive application widened its usage to include a myriad of other neurological and respiratory conditions. Applications include cardiogenic pulmonary edema [5], chronic hypoxic respiratory failure—with or without hypercapnia [6]—and as a preventative reintubation strategy for early extubation [6]. Improved survivals with less potential for adverse events has made NIV standard therapy in carefully selected patients in both acute and chronic settings. The advantages of NIV have been discussed in Table 8.1.

Table 8.1 Advantages of NIV

Advantages	Disadvantages
Easy to initiate—Does not need expert higher skills like intubation Can be placed and removed temporarily No need for sedation No risk of injury to trachea Low risk for barotrauma, hypotension, and nosocomial infections	Cannot be used if patient is not conscious Cannot be used for prolonged period due to risk of pressure sores and skin rashes Can cause claustrophobia

General Principles of Ventilation

Prior to a proper understanding of non-invasive ventilation, it is essential to review the basics of ventilation. Breathing is the movement of air into and out of the lungs. The principal purpose of breathing is to deliver oxygen to the respiratory system and pave the way for subsequent diffusion into the blood and to remove carbon dioxide from the body. Gas flows from high (atmospheric) pressure into the lower pressure respiratory tract and to the alveoli and vice versa. Spontaneous breathing and diffusion is a complex coordinated system of different functional units that include an intact brainstem, phrenic and related nerves that innervate the diaphragm and other muscles of respiration, a stable thoracic cage, patent airways, lung parenchyma, interstitium, capillary blood supply backed up by adequate cardiac output, and an availability of air (gas). When one or more of these units become suboptimal, respiratory failure can occur requiring mechanical assistance that could be emergent in certain situations. Crucial to the understanding of airflow distribution is the pressure gradient required in the conducting system, i.e., mouth/nose, terminal bronchioles proximal to the respiratory unit. *Transpulmonary pressure* is the difference in pressure inside the lungs (intra-alveolar) and outside the lungs (intrapleural). The movement of air is dependent on this gradient. It can be determined by multiplying airway pressure by the ratio of lung parenchyma elastance and total lung elastance for a given pressure. It is also dependent on airway resistance. Airway resistance is proportional to the radius of the airway. Pressure in the smaller airways contributes more to this pressure than the pressure in the larger ones. Pleural pressure, normally slightly positive during resting states, can be severely elevated in conditions like pneumothorax, effusion, any intra-abdominal condition that forces the diaphragm cephalad (e.g., pregnancy, ascites, intra-abdominal sepsis, etc.) and also with obesity. Esophageal catheters exist that can be used to determine the extent that these processes are contributing to patient condition. With spontaneous breathing, as the chest wall expands due to the contraction of the diaphragm and the respiratory muscles, negative pressure is created in the pleural space that contributes to the change in transpulmonary pressure. Older negative pressure ventilators like the iron lung and the chest cuirass or "turtle shell" artificially reproduced this mechanism to assist with breathing. In contrast, positive pressure ventilators supply gas to the respiratory unit by creating positive pressure in the proximal airways that force gas into the distal airways. Since airway resistance is radius dependent, the propelled gas is distributed unequally. This means that portions of lower resistance enjoy a greater share.

Brief Overview of Mechanical Ventilation

Though original ventilators were designed for this very basic purpose, they were quite primitive. First-generation ventilators provided mainly volume control modes without patient triggering. This required large amounts of sedation—often in conjunction with a neuromuscular blocking agent to prevent patient effort. Second-generation ventilators allowed for patient triggering and had basic built in alarms, while third-generation ventilators were microprocessor controlled, were markedly more responsive, and had extensive alarms and monitoring. Currently, fourth-generation ventilators have evolved to include a plethora of additional functional capabilities, modes, and synchronization options designed for maximal patient comfort. Most current generation ventilators also include "smart" or "closed loop" modes that adjust settings based on feedback generated from the patient and fed back to the ventilator. One newer mode now available for use, NAVA (Neurally Adjusted Ventilatory Assist), uses a transesophageal catheter to sense phrenic nerve impulse and delivers the ventilator breath in proportion and in synchrony to the neural diaphragmatic signal. Interestingly, NAVA comes equipped with a specially designed non-invasive enhancement. Although new and lacking solid evidence for their use, companies are designing and manufacturing machines with modes and options that are increasingly responsive to patient demand and able to adapt and change to ensure optimal patient/machine synchrony. These machines have been especially helpful in delivering NIV. Prone to leaks, auto triggering and dyssynchrony modern ventilator technologies—many with specific NIV options—alleviate many of these factors.

How Does a Ventilator Work?

A basic positive pressure ventilator would use a hand operated pump with a piston and compressor that drives gas into the patient's airways through a mask or a tracheal tube. The advanced variation of this system would incorporate a self-inflating power driven pump. The power could be electric, pneumatic or use a combined source. The pump is connected to the interface through a circuit that includes a one-way valve permitting the movement of gas from the ventilator to the patient. When the pump is compressed, it would allow airflow from the patient to the atmosphere as the ventilator pump inflates [7]. With these basic primary functions, the operator can set the volume of gas delivered with each breath, the respiratory rate, the timing of delivery, the flow rate at which the breath is delivered, and the fraction of oxygen in the delivered gas. Depending on patient demand, the breath could be "controlled," or "assisted" with either pressure or volume. Both inspiratory and expiratory times would be adjusted according to patient physiology, demand, and respiratory time constants. A spontaneous breath is patient initiated and can be augmented with volume or pressure. A controlled or mandatory breath is delivered when spontaneous breathing is absent. Mode of ventilation refers to a specific pattern of ventilation—either spontaneous or controlled. Over the years, endless variations of these basic modes have appeared with vast nomenclature and their discussion is beyond the scope of this chapter.

Breath Delivery

As mentioned earlier, gas is delivered either via a preset pressure or a preset volume. With the former, the operator sets the desired pressure and volume varies. With the latter, pressure varies but volumes are constant. The most important function of the ventilator is to deliver a volume of gas (tidal volume) with every breath. Other variables like flow rate and inspiratory times can also be manipulated by the clinician. The reader should understand that with pressure controlled breaths, flow fluctuates and is dependent on lung characteristics. Conversely when the operator controls the volume and flow, the inspiratory pressure can vary breath to breath. The signal that begins the breath is called the trigger variable and the one that ends inspiration being the limit variable. The variant that ends inspiration is termed the cycle variable. Factors that can initiate inspiration are (a) Time—(in controlled ventilation) when the operator sets the respiratory rate (b) Pressure and/or Flow—when the ventilator senses either a drop in pressure or a reversal in flow from patient effort. These triggers can be manually set by the operator or preset by the manufacturer [8]. The maximum levels these variables can be set are referred to as limit variables. Like the trigger variables, these limits can also be manually set by the operator or preset by the manufacturer. Finally, breath cycle termination can be determined by time, flow, pressure, or volume. The operator should consider all these variables, patient characteristics, and the goals of ventilation before selecting a particular mode of ventilation to ensure maximum patient/ventilator synchrony and comfort.

Basic Definitions in Mechanical Ventilation

Understanding the mechanics of ventilation requires knowledge of some basic terms that are used in mechanical ventilation. We have explained some of the commonly used terms as below.

Positive End Expiratory Pressure (PEEP): The supra-atmospheric pressure that exists in the alveoli at the end of expiration is PEEP. Physiologic or intrinsic PEEP is considered to be about 3–5 cmH$_2$O. This end expiratory pressure assists in preventing airway collapse and alveolar compromise and thus supports oxygenation. Higher "intrinsic" PEEP (Auto-PEEP) develops when expiration is incomplete and often occurs in those with obstructive lung diseases. A variety of strategies exist to alleviate auto-PEEP experienced during mechanical ventilation. These include but are not limited to bronchodilator therapy if warranted, adequate suctioning and appropriate airway size, shortening inspiratory time and rate, and by increasing the extrinsic or set PEEP. Auto-PEEP can make triggering of the ventilator difficult causing dyssynchrony and wasted patient effort and every attempt should be made to minimize its effects. Along with improved oxygenation and the potential for less dyssynchrony, there is evidence that PEEP may also support left ventricular function in some. *Continuous Positive Airway Pressure (CPAP)*—same as PEEP but without added inspiratory support—is now a frontline treatment used by first responders to treat those with acute congestive heart failure and pulmonary edema [9]. It is frequently used to treat obstructive sleep apnea (OSA) by alleviating or ameliorating upper airway collapse that occurs during sleep. Aside from the benefits, potential detrimental effects of PEEP and CPAP include decreased venous return and cardiac output and the potential for cerebral hypoperfusion from increased intrathoracic pressure—especially in patients with raised intracranial pressures [10].

Peak Pressure: The highest airway pressure that occurs during an active inspiration is called the peak pressure. Peak pressure is the end result of both resistance and compliance and is elevated with a variety of conditions. Factors relating to increased airway resistance and/or decreased lung compliance can cause increased peak pressures. Bronchospasm (increased resistance) and pneumothorax (decreased compliance) both result in an increase in peak pressure. Other situations such as with intra-abdominal pathologies, chest wall edema, and obesity can also result in an increase in peak ventilator pressures.

Plateau pressure: Plateau pressure is used as a surrogate for alveolar pressure and is measured by utilizing a breath hold at the end of inspiration. Higher plateau pressures are measured in conditions with poor lung compliance like Acute Respiratory Distress Syndrome [11] (ARDS). Plateau pressures ≥ 30 cmH$_2$O are associated with higher mortality in those with ARDS [11] and have been linked to increased incidence of Ventilator Induced Lung Injury (VILI)—a condition that mimics ARDS—in those with normal lung function [12].

Tidal volume and Minute ventilation: The volume of gas that is delivered to the lung with each breath is called tidal volume. Minute ventilation is the amount of gas that is delivered to the lungs every 60 s. Hence minute ventilation is equal to the product of the tidal volume and the respiratory rate. Normal minute ventilation is 4–6 lpm. Higher minute volume is often the result of increased metabolic demand as with sepsis.

Non-invasive Ventilation (NIV)

Non-invasive ventilation is a lifesaving therapy that, as mentioned prior, could avoid complications associated with invasive positive pressure ventilation (IPPV). It's imperative however that this is done in the right clinical setting and in carefully selected patients. As gas is delivered with NIV to the patient via a tight fitting facial mask, nasal mask, "helmet," or other interface without the need of an invasive tracheal tube, the goals of NIV should be clearly established prior to initiating it. The operator should also be aware of the relative contraindications of NIV (discussed later). Good evidence exists for the use of NIV with acute respiratory failure caused by various clinical conditions [Table 8.2]. These include Chronic Obstructive Pulmonary Disease (COPD) exacerbations, bronchial asthma, pulmonary edema, infections like pneumonia—with or without hypercapnia—and also in chronic respiratory failure from neurological conditions, sleep disordered breathing and with hypercapnic COPD [13]. It has also been used with success as a bridge to earlier liberation from invasive mechanical ventilation [14]. NIV is considered standard care in milder forms of both hypoxic and hypercapnic respiratory failure and guidelines have been established for its implementation.

Basic Definitions in NIV

Inspiratory Positive Airway Pressure: The amount of pressure above atmospheric pressure maintained in the airway during the inspiratory phase of breathing. By

Table 8.2 Flowchart regarding NIPPV initiation and management

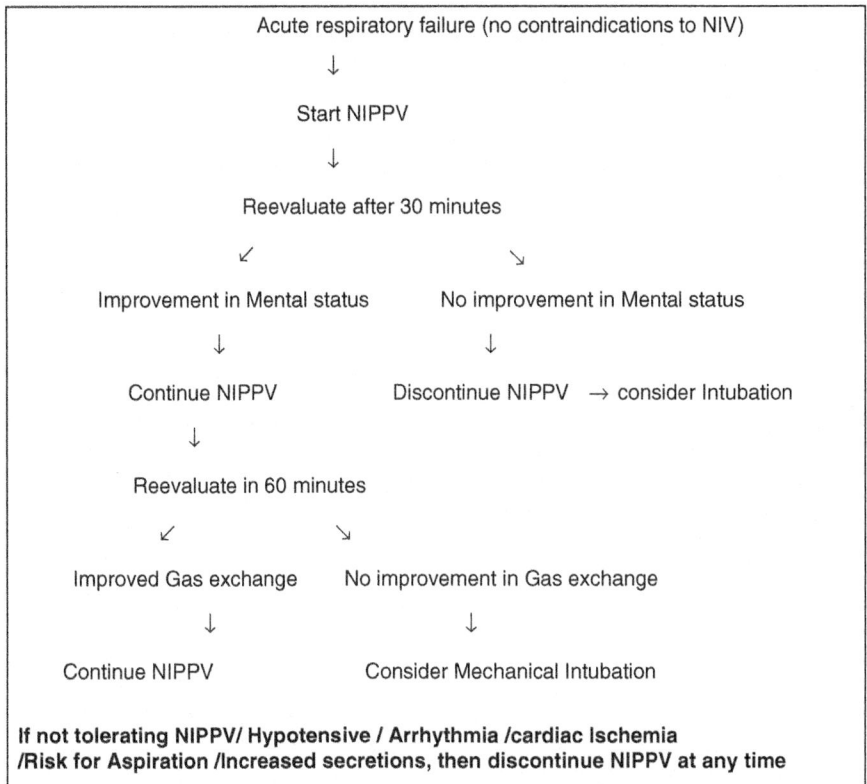

definition, the difference between the IPAP and EPAP (*see below*) constitutes the inspiratory or pressure support provided to the patient during ventilation.

Expiratory Positive Airway Pressure: The amount of pressure above atmospheric pressure maintained in the airways during the expiratory phase of breathing is coined EPAP, thus it is synonymous with PEEP and CPAP.

Ventilator Modes in NIV

The choice of a particular mode in NIV depends on the condition that is being treated, the extent of respiratory failure, and the presence or absence of hypercarbia along with patient characteristics. In this section, we will discuss the common modes of non-invasive ventilation. Most patients are ventilated with pressure targeted ventilators, though volume targeted ventilators are commercially available for providing NIV. The pressure targeted ventilators are limited by pressure and triggered and cycled by flow or time. They deliver gas and work to improve the minute ventilation by providing an IPAP and an EPAP. Three common modes—Continuous

Positive Airway Pressure (CPAP), Bi-level Positive Airway pressure (BPAP), and Average Volume Assured Pressure Support (AVAPS)—will be briefly discussed here. The other modes are less commonly used and readers are encouraged to independently research the literature for a better understanding.

CPAP: With CPAP ventilation, the same pressure—above atmospheric—is maintained both during inspiration and expiration. Thus the IPAP and EPAP are the same in this mode. The patient is able to breathe spontaneously at the set pressure and has control over the rate as well as the depth of breathing. The breathing can be more "controlled" if the operator sets a minimum and/or a maximum pressure that varies with the patient's respiratory characteristics. This mode is commonly used in acute and chronic hypoxic respiratory failure as well as with OSA.

BPAP mode: This mode uses pressure targeted ventilation and utilizes different pressures during inspiration and expiration. The IPAP is the reflection of the pressure support provided by the ventilator and is the pressure set above the EPAP. A wider gradient between IPAP and EPAP delivers a higher inspiratory pressure. This is the most commonly used mode and is very useful in the treatment of hypercapnic respiratory failure.

AVAPS mode: This mode incorporates a targeted tidal volume that is achieved by allowing the clinician to set a range in pressure or volume targets. Setting a fixed pressure support level does not allow the machine to take into account changes in patient dynamics, characteristics or for changes in the compliance of the lung, the resistance of the airways, and for patient effort during the breath. AVAPS is useful in treating many neuromuscular conditions as well as with chronic hypoventilation syndromes that cause respiratory failure. Moreover, AVAPS combined with BPAP has been successfully used in the treatment of acute hypercapnic respiratory failure [15].

NIV in Ambulatory Care

The general indications of NIV are present in Table 8.3. The commercial availability of portable ventilators has made it possible to utilize them outside of the critical care arena. Patients with chronic stable hypoxic and/or hypercapnic respiratory failure, from a variety of lung pathologies, neuromuscular diseases and hypoventilations syndromes from obstructive sleep apnea or obesity benefit the most [16]. Clear evidence exists demonstrating that use of NIV in these patients results in increased activity levels, improved oxygenation and acid base balance, with improved survival and quality of life [17]. Thus NIV is a cost-effective way of delivering life sustaining therapy and is likely to divert resources and save hospital beds for patients that need hospital admission. Ambulatory NIV tends to be more comfortable and less restrictive to patients when they are allowed to receive their care in a familiar environment. However, the prevailing limitation with home-based ventilator therapy is the poor monitoring and scarcity of properly trained personnel to operate the ventilators. This is partially overcome by training patients and their family members to care for the ventilators and to properly clean the accessories. Despite that, it remains quite a challenge to care for all of the complex needs of one that requires this level of care.

Table 8.3 Indications for NIPPV

Acute respiratory failure
Chronic obstructive pulmonary disease (COPD) exacerbation
Bronchial asthma exacerbation
Acute pulmonary edema
Pneumonia
Chronic respiratory failure from neurological conditions
Obstructive sleep apnea/sleep-related hypoventilation
Chronic COPD
Invasive mechanical ventilation weaning

Complications and Contraindications for NIV

The complication profile of NIV is much different than invasive ventilation although there are overlaps. NIV clearly avoids injury to the vocal cords, tracheal stenosis, and the need for increased sedation requirements. The ability to remove the interface for periods of time allows for the possibility of speech and diet as well. Although ventilator-associated nosocomial infections, barotrauma, and hypotension from reduced cardiac output can occur with NIV, they are less common. Pressure sores and skin rashes from device interface and claustrophobia are frequent reasons for noncompliance. Aspiration and airway obstruction should be expected and require both careful patient selection and close monitoring. Immediate removal of the mask and commencement of appropriate treatment is required with complications. Airway clearance techniques along with cough assistance may be beneficial in the prevention of aspiration and mucus plugging. Pneumothorax [18], pneumomediastinum, and pneumocephalus [19] from positive pressure are uncommon but can occur and could be life-threatening. It is always prudent to carefully consider whether the patient is appropriate for NIV prior to initiating it.

In general, any condition that necessitates emergent intubation is an absolute contraindication for NIV. Thus respiratory arrest, severe sepsis with shock, critical acidosis, hypotension, low Glasgow Coma Scale, active upper GI bleed, and severe neuromuscular weakness with inability to trigger the ventilator or clear respiratory secretions should be avoided. When possible, patient contribution, understanding, and preference about the use of NIV should be discussed prior to initiation. [20]

Conclusion

Non-invasive ventilation is an effective alternative to invasive ventilation in carefully selected patients and can be performed in both inpatient and outpatient settings. Neuromuscular disease leading to chronic respiratory failure is a frequent indication for NIV and should be considered in all patients who require assisted ventilation. Though complications occur, there is an established overall survival benefit for these patients.

Key Points

1. Non-invasive ventilation (NIV) is defined as the provision of respiratory support to patients with respiratory failure without invasive means such as with an endotracheal or tracheostomy tube.

    Non-invasive ventilators deliver positive pressure through a snug fitting mask, nasal pillows, or a variety of other interfaces rather than an artificial tube.
2. NIV is considered standard care in milder forms of both hypoxic and hypercapnic respiratory failure and guidelines have been established for its implementation.
3. *Transpulmonary pressure* is the difference in pressure inside the lungs (intra-alveolar) and outside the lungs (intrapleural).
4. The volume of gas that is delivered to the lung with each breath is called tidal volume. Minute ventilation is the amount of gas that is delivered to the lungs every 60 s.
5. *Continuous Positive Airway Pressure (CPAP)*—same as PEEP but without added inspiratory support—is now a frontline treatment used by first responders to treat those with acute congestive heart failure and pulmonary edema.
6. NIV is a cost-effective way of delivering life sustaining therapy and is likely to divert resources and save hospital beds for patients that need hospital admission.
7. In general, any condition that necessitates emergent intubation is an absolute contraindication for NIV. Thus in respiratory arrest, severe sepsis with shock, critical acidosis, hypotension, low Glasgow Coma Scale, active upper GI bleed, and severe neuromuscular weakness with inability to trigger the ventilator or clear respiratory secretions, NIV should be avoided.

References

1. Davis JE, Sternbach GL, Varon J. Paracelsus and mechanical ventilation. Resuscitation. 2000;47(1):3–5.
2. Dalziel J. On sleep and apparatus for promoting artificial respiration. Br Assoc Adv Sci. 1838;1:127.
3. Drinker P, Shaw LA. An apparatus for the prolonged administration of artificial respiration: I A design for adults and children. J Clin Invest. 1929;7:229–47.
4. http://www.washingtontimes.com/news/2014/aug/24/north-texan-one-of-10-still-living-in-iron-lung/.
5. Gray A, Goodacre S, Newby D, et al. Noninvasive ventilation in acute cardiogenic pulmonary edema. NEJM. 2008;359:142–51.
6. Brochard L, Isabey D, Piquet J, et al. Reversal of acute exacerbations of chronic obstructive lung disease by inspiratory assistance with a face mask. NEJM. 1990;323:1523–30.
7. Chatburn RL. A new system for understanding mechanical ventilators. Respir Care. 1991;36:1123.
8. Chatburn RL. Classification of mechanical ventilators. Respir Care. 1992;37:1009.
9. Peter JV, Moran JL, Phillips-Hughes J, et al. Effect of non-invasive positive pressure ventilation (NIPPV) on mortality in patients with acute cardiogenic pulmonary edema, a meta-analysis. Lancet. 367:1155–63.

10. Marik P, Chen K, Varon J, et al. Management of acute intracranial hypertension: a review for clinicians. J Emerg Med. 1999;17(4):711–9.
11. Amato MB, Meade MO, Slutsky AS, et al. Driving pressure and survival in the acute respiratory distress syndrome. N Engl J Med. 2015;372(8):747–55.
12. Presenti A. Target blood gases during ARDS ventilator management (editorial). Intensive Care Med. 1990;16(6):3449–51.
13. Elliot MW, Mulvey DA, Moxham J, et al. Domiciliary nocturnal nasal intermittent positive pressure ventilation in COPD: mechanisms underlying changes in arterial blood gas tensions. Eur Respir J. 1991;4:1044.
14. Adıyeke E, Ozgultekin A, Turan G, et al. Non-invasive mechanical ventilation after the successful weaning: a comparison with the venturi mask. Braz J Anesthesiol. 2016;66(6):572–6.
15. Briones Claudett KH, Briones Claudett M, Chung Sang Wong M, et al. Noninvasive mechanical ventilation with average volume assured pressure support (AVAPS) in patients with chronic obstructive pulmonary disease and hypercapnic encephalopathy. BMC Pulm Med. 2013;13:12.
16. Mehta S, Gill NS. Noninvasive ventilation. Am J Respir Crit Care Med. 2001;163:540–77.
17. Leger P, Jennequin J, Gerard M, et al. Home positive pressure ventilation via nasal mask for patients with neuromusculoskeletal disorders. Respir Care. 1989;7:640s–4s.
18. Simmonds A. Pneumothorax; an important complication of non-invasive ventilation in neuromuscular disease. Neuromuscul Disord. 2004;4(6):351–2.
19. Nair SR, Henry MT. Pneumocephalus induced by non-invasive ventilation; a case report. Respir Med Extra. 2005;1:75–7.
20. Gregoretti C, Pisani L, Cortegiani A, et al. Noninvasive ventilation in critically ill patients. Crit Care Clin. 2015;31(3):435–57.

Non-invasive Ventilation in NeuroMuscular Diseases

Hariharan Regunath, Troy Whitacre, and Stevan P. Whitt

Introduction

Neuromuscular diseases (NMDs) result from congenital or acquired disorders of the spinal cord, motor nerves, neuromuscular junction or muscles, and occasionally from anatomical abnormalities that cause mechanical ineffectiveness despite otherwise normal tissue. Acute and chronic NMDs cause weakness of respiratory and airway muscles, which is often progressive, and often culminates in respiratory failure, which is the leading cause of death in these patients [1–3]. A clear understanding of the functional anatomy of the respiratory system coupled with an understanding of the underlying pathophysiology and rate of progression of the neuromuscular diseases is essential to selection of an appropriate ventilator support strategy and determination of prognosis [3]. Ventilatory interventions may prevent complications, and therefore improve morbidity and mortality in patients with NMDs [4]. With the increased awareness of nocturnal hypoventilation in patients with NMDs, use of nocturnal non-invasive ventilation (NIV) has gained impetus [4–6]. NIV can also be used for carefully selected NMDs episodically, for example following aspiration, lower respiratory tract infection, or myasthenic

---

H. Regunath, M.D. (✉)
Divisions of Pulmonary, Critical Care and Infectious Diseases,
Department of Medicine, University of Missouri, Columbia, MO, USA
e-mail: regunathh@health.missouri.edu

T. Whitacre, R.R.T.
Respiratory Therapy Services, University of Missouri Hospital and Clinics,
Columbia, MO, USA
e-mail: whitacret@health.missouri.edu

S. P. Whitt, M.D.
Division of Pulmonary, Critical Care and Environmental Medicine,
Department of Medicine, University of Missouri, Columbia, MO, USA
e-mail: whitts@health.missouri.edu

crisis, provided their upper airway remains patent and intact [7]. In this chapter we provide an overview of NIV in NMDs, relevant pathophysiology of respiratory failure in NMDs and discuss available evidence of appropriate NIV use for patients with specific NMDs.

Neurophysiology of Respiratory Function

Ventilation is primarily an involuntary process regulated by the brainstem, but voluntary control can be achieved by signals from the cerebral cortex [8]. At rest, inspiration is an active process, whereas expiration is largely passive recoil of the thorax to functional residual lung capacity (FRC). Neurons in the medullary respiratory center discharge impulses periodically to the cervical and thoracic spinal cord, and from there, relayed to the muscles of respiration. Complex feedback mechanisms, comprising chemical and mechanical receptors, modulate involuntary control centers. These chemoreceptors sense changes in pH, arterial partial pressure of carbon dioxide ($PaCO_2$) [central chemoreceptors], and arterial partial pressure of oxygen (PaO_2) [peripheral chemoreceptors]. Mechanoreceptors sense pulmonary stretch (Hering–Breuer reflex) [8]. Figure 9.1 is a schematic representation of neurologic control of respiratory mechanics.

Classification of Neuromuscular Diseases

NMDs can be classified as follows, and are categorized in Table 9.1 [3, 9, 10].

1. Site of neuraxial affection: Spinal cord, neuropathic, neuromuscular junction, and myopathic.
2. Disease onset: Acute or chronic.

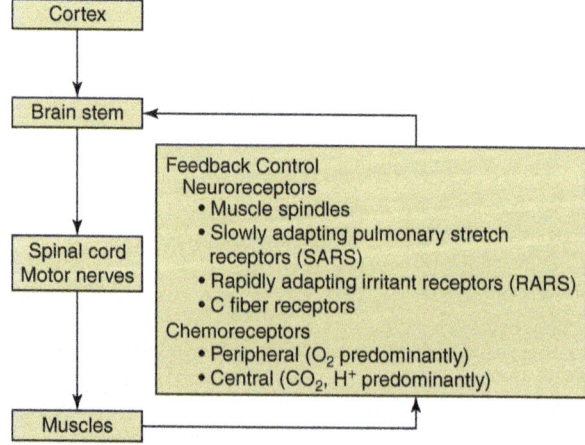

Fig. 9.1 Neurochemical control of respiratory function (Reprinted from Murray and Nadel's Textbook of Respiratory Medicine, Vol 97, Sixth Edition, Joshua O Benditt and F. Dennis McCool, Respiratory System and Neuromuscular Diseases, 1691–1706.e4, Copyright © 2016, 2010, 2005 by Saunders, an imprint of Elsevier Inc. with permission from Elsevier)

Table 9.1 Neuromuscular diseases causing respiratory dysfunction

Onset	Spinal cord/neuropathic disorders	Neuromuscular junction disorders	Myopathic disorders
Acute	• Guillain–Barre syndrome • Cervical spinal cord injury • Critical illness neuropathy • Multiple sclerosis • Transverse myelitis • Epidural abscess • Acute poliomyelitis • Paralytic rabies	• Myasthenia gravis • Lambert–Eaton myasthenic syndrome • Congenital myasthenic syndrome • Botulism • Venoms (snake, scorpions, ticks) • Neuromuscular junction blockers • Organophosphorus poisoning	
Chronic	• Spinal cord injury • Motor neuron disease • Amyotrophic lateral sclerosis • Spinal muscular atrophy • Post-polio syndrome • Chronic inflammatory demyelinating polyneuropathy • Charcot–Marie–tooth disease		• Muscular dystrophies • Myotonic dystrophy • Inflammatory myopathies • Congenital and metabolic myopathies

3. Disease progression: Slow, variable, rapidly progressive, or non-progressive.
4. Mode of acquisition: Congenital or acquired disorders.

Pathophysiology of Respiratory Failure in Neuromuscular Diseases

Hypoventilation from poor effort and resultant lung restriction (reduced compliance), inability to effectively clear respiratory secretions, and failure of upper or lower airway patency are the main mechanisms of respiratory failure in NMDs. Depending on the degree of weakness of inspiratory, expiratory, and airway muscles, the clinical manifestations and the interventions differ [2, 6]. Inspiratory muscle weakness results in atelectasis from prolonged low lung volumes and failure to clear secretions. Compensation over time results in tachypnea, but as the NMD advances, chest wall compliance is further reduced by progressive respiratory muscle atrophy, and/or spinal and other anatomical deformities [11]. This progression can overload the already fatigued respiratory muscles and worsen hypoventilation, which manifests first nocturnally, and then in advanced stages during day time, and eventually as chronic hypercapnic acidosis [6]. In addition, the limitation of lung volumes in the supine position, many times with contributions from obstructive apnea or cardiomyopathy associated with certain NMDs, predisposes to sleep disordered breathing [5]. Hypoxia is usually a late manifestation [6]. See Fig. 9.2.

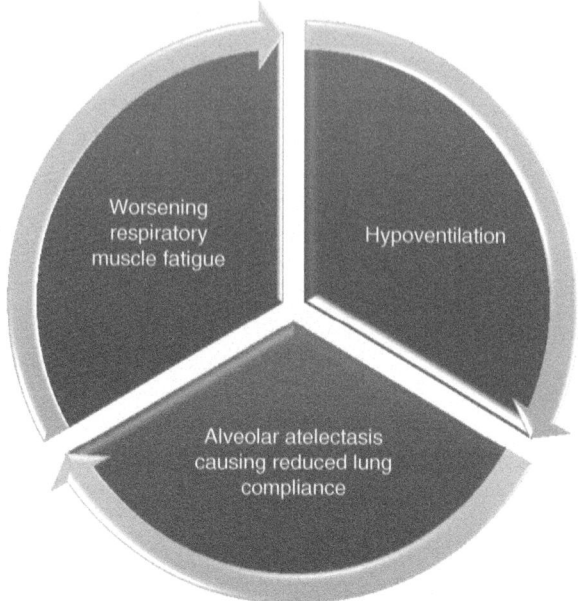

Fig. 9.2 Vicious circle of respiratory failure in neuromuscular disease

When muscles of expiration and airway (bulbar) are affected, inability to effectively clear respiratory and oral secretions result in atelectasis and aspiration, respectively [12–14].

During normal sleep, muscle tone is reduced during rapid eye movement (REM) phase along with a decline in tidal volume and respiratory rate. Moreover, the chemosensitivity of the respiratory center and activity of nerves innervating pharyngeal dilators are also reduced [5]. In health, the phrenic nerve is least affected, whereas those nerves supplying the respiratory muscles of the airway and chest wall are most suppressed. These normal physiological changes are less well tolerated by patients with coexisting NMD, and are observed as an increased susceptibility to sleep disordered breathing [5]. Early manifestations are classically described as "saw-tooth desaturations" during REM sleep, and as weakness progresses, hypoventilation results and extends into non-REM (NREM) sleep. Associated cardiomyopathies commonly add central sleep disordered breathing patterns such as Cheyne–Stokes respirations. Other clinical manifestations such as macroglossia or chest wall abnormalities can result in the development of obstructive sleep apnea [15–17].

Diagnosis of Neuromuscular Respiratory Failure

While dyspnea/tachypnea, exhaustion, diaphoresis, and the inability to speak in complete sentences are all obvious manifestations of respiratory failure, in someone with suspected NMD, such overt signs may not be present. History should focus not only respiratory symptoms, but also sleep quality, nighttime awakenings, and fatigue. Symptoms of nocturnal hypoventilation include sudden awakening from sleep, an irregular pattern of respiration while asleep, early morning frontal headache, and excessive daytime sleepiness [9]. During exam, particular focus should be on neurological assessment of the airway muscles, chest and abdominal exams, and assessment of accessory muscles of respiration. Paradoxical inward movement of the abdomen with inspiration is an ominous sign of impending respiratory failure [18]. Ocular exam may reveal ptosis or ophthalmoparesis in patients with myasthenia gravis (MG) or Guillain-Barre syndrome (GBS). Bulbar weakness can be a dominant finding in the acute phase of GBS or MG and ALS, as well as diphtheria and botulism [6] .Chest exam may reveal diminished breath sounds, crepitations, or bronchial breath sounds if atelectasis or pneumonitis is present. Bedside spirometry, blood gas testing, and imaging studies of the chest are essential diagnostic adjuncts [6].

In the presence of symptoms, NIV is indicated when any one of the following is present [19].

1. Partial pressure of carbon dioxide ($PaCO_2$) ≥ 45 mmHg
2. Nocturnal desaturation to $\leq 88\%$ for five consecutive minutes or longer
3. Maximum inspiratory pressures <60 cmH_2O or FVC $<50\%$ predicted

An elevated or rising serum bicarbonate level may be an early sign of undiagnosed nocturnal hypercapnia and has been predictive of mortality in patients with ALS [1]. In all patients with hypercapnia, it may be prudent to check thyroid stimulating hormone levels [20].

The most recent recommendation for the management of ALS patients, from the American Academy of Neurology (AAN), is nocturnal oximetry (nocturnal desaturations $<90\%$ for one cumulative minute) or measurement of maximal inspiratory pressure (<-60 cmH_2O) or both, and erect and supine forced vital capacity (FVC $<50\%$ of predicted, supine value is a better measure of diaphragm weakness). In the presence of any value less than these recommended values, NIV can be considered [1].

Non-invasive Ventilation in Neuromuscular Diseases

NIV consists of intermittent or continuous positive pressure, delivered through a mask or an interface to the nose or mouth or both [21]. The two main modes of non-invasive ventilation for use in NMDs are continuous positive airway pressure (CPAP) and bilevel positive airway pressure. Bilevel ventilation is more advantageous than CPAP, in that it provides increased pressure support during inspiration that reduces the inspiratory load on muscles, in addition to positive end-expiratory pressure (PEEP) provided by CPAP to prevent atelectasis [21]. Other potential modes include pressure support, pressure control, and newer adaptive modes of ventilation. Nasal or oronasal masks are most convenient for nocturnal ventilation [22]. Implementation of nocturnal NIV initially ameliorates the gas exchange abnormalities effectively for both night and day times. As the respiratory muscle weakness progresses, nocturnal ventilation alone becomes inadequate to control daytime respiratory failure. Daytime

NIV can be delivered using the same interface used for the night, but a convenient mouthpiece can also be substituted, according to patient preference, and is commonly referred to as sips ventilation (SV) or mouth piece ventilation (MPV) [22–25]. In recent years, home ventilation strategies have incorporated daytime ventilation via various available mouthpieces to enable intermittent positive pressure ventilation (IPPV) [4, 26, 27]. MPV provides the benefit of social convenience, avoidance of skin breakdown on the face associated with prolonged use of nasal or oronasal masks, and the preserved ability to speak and swallow. Drawbacks include less ideal seal, an increased need for patient involvement and initiative, and longer initial training for implementation [4]. There are a variety of cough assist devices which may be necessary in addition to NIV for optimal clearance of respiratory secretions, but it is beyond the scope of this chapter to discuss them in detail.

Evidence supporting the use of NIV is limited to few studies because of ethical concerns in conducting a randomized controlled trial [9, 13, 26, 28–31]. NIV has typically been helpful in slow respiratory deterioration with progressive NMDs (like amyotrophic lateral sclerosis [ALS] and muscular dystrophies) with chronic respiratory failure without bulbar affection—for both treatment and prevention of acute exacerbations [32, 33]. Other reasonable uses include acute illness such as early myasthenia crisis, where prompt initiation of NIV (bilevel) prior to the appearance of gas exchange abnormalities has been shown to avoid intubation, which is associated with prolongation of hospital stay and ventilator-associated complications. Moreover, NIV can be used for outpatient (home) ventilation [26, 28, 29, 34]. When NIV is judiciously combined with cough assist devices (mechanical and other modalities to clear airway secretions), the number and duration of hospitalizations is reduced [13, 14, 26, 28, 30]. The goals of NIV in NMDs include: [22].

1. Improve and maintain pulmonary compliance by reducing alveolar atelectasis
2. Optimize alveolar ventilation
3. Assist clearance of respiratory secretions

The use of NIV in NMDs is clearly contraindicated when there is bulbar affection or rapid progression of acute respiratory failure with quick deterioration of gas exchange, when invasive mechanical ventilation with intubation is required. The usual contraindications for NIV are as follows [7].

1. Respiratory arrest
2. Inability to protect airway
3. Severely impaired mental status (GCS of ≤ 8)
4. Inability to clear respiratory secretions with usual methods
5. Hypotension or shock
6. Massive upper gastrointestinal bleeding or actively vomiting
7. Multi-organ failure
8. Inability to fit mask

Experts have also described other additional contraindications for long-term use of NIV in NMDs such as patient noncooperation, high oxygen requirements, severe hypercapnia with acidosis, persistent hypoxia despite optimal cough assist techniques, seizures or severe agitation, conditions that interfere with fitting of the mask and inadequate support from caregivers [6, 22].

Acute phases of GBS, high cervical spinal cord injury, and other acute neuropathic/myelopathic diseases (see Table 9.1) are also considered as contraindications, but NIV combined with assisted coughing techniques can still be very helpful during the recovery phase. NIV can be useful to facilitate not only successful extubation (if dysautonomia has resolved and motor strength continues to improve) but also improved outcomes for the post-extubation period [6, 35]. Concomitant chronic obstructive pulmonary disease (COPD) and/or congestive heart failure may be another indication for successful use of NIV in NMDs [7, 21]. For cervical cord lesions below C3 level where some diaphragm function is preserved, NIV can be judiciously used for weaning based on the residual ventilatory function [22]. But, even in high spinal cord injury (C2-C3) if the following goals can be met, then full-time NIV has been suggested as an alternative for tracheostomy ventilation [22].

1. Ability to stack breaths by glossopharyngeal breathing (use of lingual muscles to gulp air followed by glottis closure to increase lung volume and peak cough flows) from a volume cycled ventilator.
2. Adequate alveolar ventilation achievable with nasal, oronasal, or mouthpiece interface
3. Patients can be educated for effective use of cough enhancing techniques to clear

In patients with ALS, favorable responses to NIV have been reported in a small prospective study in patients with preserved bulbar function and the following findings: orthopnea, daytime hypercapnia, and nocturnal desaturations [20, 36]. NIV use has been associated with a slower decline in FVC when instituted following detection of hypercapnia or development of orthopnea with MIP <60% of predicted [33]. Hence, some authors suggest earlier institution of NIV (before the development of hypercapnia) in order to provide the benefit of improved survival [20, 37].

In patients requiring NIV for both nocturnal and daytime use, scrutiny must be used to avoid potential long-term complications, which are mainly associated with the nasal or oronasal interface. Pressure-related skin damage and orthodontic deformities, oral and nasal dryness predisposing to sinusitis, and ocular irritation from air leak are reported complications [22]. Most adverse effects can be circumvented by intermittent use of the oral interface (MPV as in sips ventilation). Lack of cooperation and persistent hypoxia despite adequate use along with cough assist techniques are relative contraindications for long-term NIV use.

In summary, NIV has become a valuable initial choice for respiratory failure in select NMDs such as ALS and muscular dystrophies, both for acute phases and exacerbations of chronic phase disease. Clear understanding of indications, contraindications, and knowledge of appropriate patient selection is essential. Successful implementation requires patient education, selection of appropriate interface and ventilator settings, and close initial monitoring. In the acute setting, patients with MG derive the most benefit when NIV is implemented early in myasthenia crisis even before gas exchange abnormalities, whereas it can cause dangerous delay to definitive therapy and complications when used for those patients in the most acute phase of GBS. Ethical concerns are cited as a limiting factor to definitive randomized controlled trials of NIV in patients with NMD. Small trial and observational data, along with expert opinion, make up the lion's share of available evidence to guide use of NIV in NMDs.

Key Points

1. In patients without bulbar affection, non-invasive ventilation (NIV) can be used as an alternative to ventilation, usually via tracheostomy.
2. With the increased awareness of nocturnal hypoventilation in patients with NMDs, use of nocturnal non-invasive ventilation (NIV) has gained impetus.
3. Hypoventilation from poor effort and resultant lung restriction (reduced compliance), inability to effectively clear respiratory secretions, and failure of upper or lower airway patency are the main mechanisms of respiratory failure in neuromuscular disorders.
4. While dyspnea/tachypnea, exhaustion, diaphoresis, and the inability to speak in complete sentences are all obvious manifestations of respiratory failure, in someone with suspected NMD, such overt signs may not be always present.
5. An elevated or rising serum bicarbonate level may be an early sign of undiagnosed nocturnal hypercapnia and has been predictive of mortality in patients with ALS.
6. When NIV is judiciously combined with cough assist devices (mechanical and other modalities to clear airway secretions), the number and duration of hospitalizations is reduced.
7. Concomitant chronic obstructive pulmonary disease (COPD) and/or congestive heart failure may be another indication for successful use of NIV in neuromuscular disorders.

Conflict of Interest None.

References

1. Miller RG, Jackson CE, Kasarskis EJ, England JD, Forshew D, Johnston W, et al. Practice parameter update: the care of the patient with amyotrophic lateral sclerosis: drug, nutritional, and respiratory therapies (an evidence-based review): report of the Quality Standards Subcommittee of the American Academy of Neurology. Neurology. 2009;73(15):1218–26.
2. Benditt JO, Boitano LJ. Pulmonary issues in patients with chronic neuromuscular disease. Am J Respir Crit Care Med. 2013;187(10):1046–55.
3. Perrin C, Unterborn JN, Ambrosio CD, Hill NS. Pulmonary complications of chronic neuromuscular diseases and their management. Muscle Nerve. 2004;29(1):5–27.
4. Bach JR, Goncalves MR, Hon A, Ishikawa Y, De Vito EL, Prado F, et al. Changing trends in the management of end-stage neuromuscular respiratory muscle failure: recommendations of an international consensus. Am J Phys Med Rehabil. 2013;92(3):267–77.
5. Aboussouan LS. Sleep-disordered breathing in neuromuscular disease. Am J Respir Crit Care Med. 2015;191(9):979–89.

6. Rabinstein AA. Noninvasive ventilation for neuromuscular respiratory failure: when to use and when to avoid. Curr Opin Crit Care. 2016;22(2):94–9.
7. Gregoretti C, Pisani L, Cortegiani A, Ranieri VM. Noninvasive ventilation in critically ill patients. Crit Care Clin. 2015;31(3):435–57.
8. Barrett KE, Barman SM, Boitano S, Brooks HL. Regulation of respiration. Ganong's review of medical physiology. 25th ed. McGraw-Hill Education: New York; 2016.
9. Shneerson J, Simonds A. Noninvasive ventilation for chest wall and neuromuscular disorders. Eur Respir J. 2002;20(2):480–7.
10. Ambrosino N, Carpene N, Gherardi M. Chronic respiratory care for neuromuscular diseases in adults. Eur Respir J. 2009;34(2):444–51.
11. Papastamelos C, Panitch HB, Allen JL. Chest wall compliance in infants and children with neuromuscular disease. Am J Respir Crit Care Med. 1996;154(4 Pt 1):1045–8.
12. Poponick JM, Jacobs I, Supinski G, DiMarco AF. Effect of upper respiratory tract infection in patients with neuromuscular disease. Am J Respir Crit Care Med. 1997;156(2):659–64.
13. Tzeng AC, Bach JR. Prevention of pulmonary morbidity for patients with neuromuscular disease. Chest. 2000;118(5):1390–6.
14. Bach JR, Rajaraman R, Ballanger F, Tzeng AC, Ishikawa Y, Kulessa R, et al. Neuromuscular ventilatory insufficiency: effect of home mechanical ventilator use v oxygen therapy on pneumonia and hospitalization rates. Am J Phys Med Rehabil. 1998;77(1):8–19.
15. Lemay J, Sériès F, Sénéchal M, Maranda B, Maltais F. Unusual respiratory manifestations in two young adults with Duchenne muscular dystrophy. Can Respir J. 2012;19(1):37.
16. Renard D, Humbertclaude V, Labauge P. Macroglossia in adult Duchenne muscular dystrophy. Acta Neurol Belg. 2010;110(3):288.
17. Barbe F, Quera-Salva M, McCann C, Gajdos P, Raphael J, de Lattre J, et al. Sleep-related respiratory disturbances in patients with Duchenne muscular dystrophy. Eur Respir J. 1994;7(8):1403–8.
18. Rabinstein AA, Wijdicks EFM. Warning signs of imminent respiratory failure in neurological patients. Semin Neurol. 2003;23(1):97–104.
19. Clinical indications for noninvasive positive pressure ventilation in chronic respiratory failure due to restrictive lung disease, COPD, and nocturnal hypoventilation—a consensus conference report. Chest. 1999;116(2):521–34.
20. Ozsancak A, D'Ambrosio C, Hill NS. Nocturnal noninvasive ventilation. Chest. 2008;133(5):1275–86.
21. Nava S, Hill N. Non-invasive ventilation in acute respiratory failure. Lancet. 2009;374(9685):250–9.
22. Bach JR. Continuous noninvasive ventilation for patients with neuromuscular disease and spinal cord injury. Semin Respir Crit Care Med. 2002;23(3):283–92.
23. Bach JR, Alba AS, Saporito LR. Intermittent positive pressure ventilation via the mouth as an alternative to tracheostomy for 257 ventilator users. Chest. 1993;103(1):174–82.
24. Toussaint M, Steens M, Wasteels G, Soudon P. Diurnal ventilation via mouthpiece: survival in end-stage Duchenne patients. Eur Respir J. 2006;28(3):549–55.
25. Affeldt J. Roundtable conference on poliomyelitis equipment. New York: National Foundation for Infantile Paralysis-March of Dimes White Plains; 1953.
26. Servera E, Sancho J, Zafra MJ, Catala A, Vergara P, Marin J. Alternatives to endotracheal intubation for patients with neuromuscular diseases. Am J Phys Med Rehabil. 2005;84(11):851–7.
27. Toussaint M, Chatwin M, Soudon P. Mechanical ventilation in Duchenne patients with chronic respiratory insufficiency: clinical implications of 20 years published experience. Chron Respir Dis. 2007;4(3):167–77.
28. Rabinstein A, Wijdicks EF. BiPAP in acute respiratory failure due to myasthenic crisis may prevent intubation. Neurology. 2002;59(10):1647–9.
29. Vianello A, Bevilacqua M, Arcaro G, Gallan F, Serra E. Non-invasive ventilatory approach to treatment of acute respiratory failure in neuromuscular disorders. A comparison with endotracheal intubation. Intensive Care Med. 2000;26(4):384–90.

30. Vianello A, Corrado A, Arcaro G, Gallan F, Ori C, Minuzzo M, et al. Mechanical insufflation-exsufflation improves outcomes for neuromuscular disease patients with respiratory tract infections. Am J Phys Med Rehabil. 2005;84(2):83–8; discussion 9–91.
31. Aboussouan LS, Khan SU, Meeker DP, Stelmach K, Mitsumoto H. Effect of noninvasive positive-pressure ventilation on survival in amyotrophic lateral sclerosis. Ann Intern Med. 1997;127(6):450–3.
32. McKim DA, Road J, Avendano M, Abdool S, Cote F, Duguid N, et al. Home mechanical ventilation: a Canadian Thoracic Society clinical practice guideline. Can Respir J. 2011;18(4):197–215.
33. Bourke SC, Tomlinson M, Williams TL, Bullock RE, Shaw PJ, Gibson GJ. Effects of non-invasive ventilation on survival and quality of life in patients with amyotrophic lateral sclerosis: a randomised controlled trial. Lancet Neurol. 2006;5(2):140–7.
34. Seneviratne J, Mandrekar J, Wijdicks EF, Rabinstein AA. Noninvasive ventilation in myasthenic crisis. Arch Neurol. 2008;65(1):54–8.
35. Bach JR, Gonçalves MR, Hamdani I, Winck JC. Extubation of patients with neuromuscular weakness: a new management paradigm. Chest. 2010;137(5):1033–9.
36. Bourke SC, Bullock RE, Williams TL, Shaw PJ, Gibson GJ. Noninvasive ventilation in ALS: indications and effect on quality of life. Neurology. 2003;61(2):171–7.
37. Lechtzin N, Scott Y, Busse AM, Clawson LL, Kimball R, Wiener CM. Early use of non-invasive ventilation prolongs survival in subjects with ALS. Amyotroph Lateral Scler. 2007;8(3):185–8.

Trouble Shooting with Noninvasive Ventilation

10

Vijay Kodadhala and Pradeep C. Bollu

Introduction

Twenty-four percent of the US population has a diagnosis of OSA; however, only about 4% carry the diagnosis [1]. Although CPAP is an extremely effective treatment for OSA, compliance is a critical problem and is widely recognized as a significant limiting factor in successful treatment [2]. Research shows that 30–50% of patients diagnosed with OSA reject CPAP immediately and approximately 80% of OSA patients are noncompliant within a year after starting CPAP therapy [3]. Noncompliance with CPAP significantly reduces the overall effectiveness of treatment of OSA, leaving these patients at an increased risk for complications associated with untreated sleep apnea with impaired daily functioning and decreased quality of life [4]. Improvement of CPAP compliance will positively impact patients, patient's families, communities, and the health care system as a whole [6, 7]. Several recent studies have confirmed varying rates of PAP adherence ranging 30–84% [10].

With the increase in awareness of sleep apnea, there is a corresponding increase in the number of patients who are diagnosed with sleep apnea and who are receiving PAP therapy which is considered as primary treatment in sleep apnea treatment. Increase in awareness regarding sleep apnea is a very positive change, as untreated sleep apnea can lead to threefold increase in risk for hypertension, diabetes mellitus, and stroke [5], increase in risk for ischemic heart disease, cardiac arrhythmia, congestive heart failure, peripheral vascular disease, and valvular cardiac disease [6], excessive daytime sleepiness, impaired cognition and memory, decreased functional and occupational capacity as well as mood alterations, all of which significantly

---

V. Kodadhala, M.D.
Fellow in Pulmonary Medicine, Howard University Hospital, Washington, DC, USA
e-mail: vkodadhala@gmail.com

P. C. Bollu, M.D. (✉)
Department of Neurology, University of Missouri, Columbia, MO, USA
e-mail: BolluP@health.missouri.edu

decrease quality of life [7]. Untreated sleep apnea patients are seven times more likely to have motor vehicle accidents and injuries than patients without the diagnosis, costing up to 16 billion dollars per year [8].

Sleep apnea patients are 2–3 times more likely to have an occupational injury or accident, which further contributes to decreased occupational productivity and increased health costs. Besides affecting the patient's quality of life and health outcomes, it has been shown that untreated OSA patients have up to two times greater health care costs than similar individuals without OSA [9].

Untreated OSA increases burden on both patient's family and also on community. It has a negative effect on the patient's bed partner's health status, sleep quality, daytime alertness, mood, overall quality of life as well as his/her personal relationship with the patient [7]. Likewise, untreated sleep apnea also affects the health care system as a whole. As previously reported, various studies have estimated the health-related cost burden of untreated sleep apnea in the United States to be approximately 3.4 billion dollars per year [9]. These astronomical costs are typically a result of more frequent practitioner visits, increased hospitalizations, and development of comorbid conditions [9].

Optimum treatment of sleep apnea with PAP therapy can result in improvement in sleep efficiency and reduction in daytime sleepiness. This can significantly impact work productivity during the daytime in a positive way. Another positive impact of daytime alertness is a reduction in potential traffic accidents, as drowsiness while driving is a well-studied cause of traffic accidents [11]. Compliant and consistent usage of PAP therapy is very important to gain full benefits that a patient can reap with PAP usage.

Several factors can result in poor PAP therapy compliance. Awareness and management of these problems that a patient may encounter while using PAP therapy can result in a significant improvement of patient's compliance. In this chapter, we will focus on day-to-day challenges a patient may encounter while using PAP therapy and simple measures that can be undertaken to alleviate these challenges. We also hope that this knowledge will help a patient to overcome such day-to-day challenges while using PAP therapy and thereby significantly improve PAP therapy adherence.

Different patients may encounter different challenges as every patient is unique. Challenges could arise from any of the components of the PAP machine. PAP machines have different parts such as a mask interface that either covers the mouth or face or just the nose depending on the type of interface used, tubes that connect the mask interface to the PAP machine, humidification chamber that adds humidity to the air that is delivered by the PAP machine, and the PAP machine itself. Another important challenge is pressure intolerance.

Any of these PAP device parts can cause discomfort or trouble to the patient, resulting in reduction in PAP therapy compliance. It is very important to adequately educate the patient about PAP therapy. Education should start when a decision is made to conduct a sleep study and should be continued until the final decision regarding treatment options is made; if PAP therapy is chosen as a mode of treatment, education should continue thereafter also. Once the patient is sufficiently educated about using PAP therapy and its common challenges, she/he will be more likely to be willing to try the treatment.

As described earlier, challenges can be in any form, either due to pressure intolerance, the machine itself, tubing, humidifier, or the mask. In this chapter, we will try to address the common problems encountered and the potential remedial actions.

Pressure Challenges

One of the important goals of any form of treatment for sleep apnea is to keep airway patent. PAP therapy is one of the treatment modalities to keep airway patent during the sleep. Depending on the severity of sleep apnea, patients may require higher pressures to keep their airways patent. This can be very challenging especially when tried for the first time, which usually is on first night of the PAP titration study. Usually, PAP titration starts with "continuous positive airway pressure" (CPAP). When patients can't tolerate high CPAP during the titration night, per protocol, CPAP can be switched to a bi-level PAP therapy which may be better tolerated.

One of the main challenges a patient may face is inability or difficulty to fall asleep due to high pressure airflow along with the added difficulty of exhaling against high pressures. There are several methods that can be tried to overcome the pressure intolerance.

1. For patients who cannot fall asleep due to high PAP pressures, starting PAP therapy at a lower pressure setting and ramping up to target pressure over a period of 30–45 min will help the patient fall asleep. If patient wakes up during the night for any reason, using this method will help the patient to go back to sleep. Most of the machines are equipped with this feature and all it takes is patient education. Patients, who are experiencing this challenge, can also call their DME (durable medical equipment) provider and inquire if this feature is available on their PAP device.
2. Another feature PAP devices typically offer is the "FLEX pressure" option. This is an exhalation relief setting. Once this feature is activated the pressure delivered by the machine will automatically be lowered during exhalation period, depending on the settings chosen. With this feature, patients can decrease the PAP pressure during their own exhalation depending on their comfort. The maximum pressure that can be lowered when compared to inspiratory pressure is 3 mmHg. This can help the patient to exhale comfortably against the low pressure and thus may improve PAP tolerance and adherence.

    Some patients may not tolerate high pressures initially. But most people tolerate high pressures over a period of time. For such patients, it is advisable to start PAP therapy with a pressure they can tolerate instead of trying to treat the sleep apnea completely right away, and gradually increasing the pressure over a period

of months to the target pressure. This will give the patient an opportunity to get adjusted to high pressures gradually.
3. In approximately 56–75% of patients with obstructive sleep apnea (OSA), the frequency and duration of apneas are influenced by body position. This is referred to as position-dependent OSA or POSA [12]. Surrounding the upper airways is soft tissue and musculature which do not have adequate support to prevent collapsing of upper airways. Muscle tone will decrease during sleep. This decreased muscle tone in addition to gravitational forces acting on pharyngeal and on the tongue musculature in supine position can lead to upper airway narrowing. Treating the sleep apnea with PAP therapy both in supine and side sleep usually requires higher PAP pressure. This is very important in patients with higher pressure intolerance because such patients can benefit from combination therapy of both PAP and positional therapy. In patients with intolerance of higher pressure settings, apnea during supine sleep can be alleviated with positional therapy with avoidance of supine sleep with positional therapy device and apnea in side sleep can be alleviated with low PAP pressure. By using the combination therapy, sleep apnea can be treated with low PAP pressure setting.

    Another form of positional therapy is elevation of head end of the bed (HOB). Elevating head of the bed itself can result in decreased collapsibility of upper air ways collapsibility. Elevating HOB just by 30–45° itself will decrease severity of sleep apnea by 25–30% [13]. Thus with the elevation of HOB, these patients will typically require low pressure to alleviate OSA. This can be adopted in patients who have pressure intolerance to higher PAP pressure. So combination of head of the bed elevation and PAP therapy is another form of combination therapy to alleviate OSA.

    For patients who can't tolerate any form of pressure, combination of mandibular advancement devices (oral appliance devices) and positional therapy is another treatment of option. Mandibular advancement devices may also be considered if the patient can't tolerate higher pressures as the combination of MAD and low CPAP pressures may be all it takes to correct their OSA.

    Although combination therapies may not be fully effective in alleviating apnea patients with severe OSA, they will at least decrease the severity of sleep apnea.
4. Aerophagia or air swallowing is another challenge a patient can encounter due to PAP therapy. This can occur both with high and low CPAP pressures. It is more commonly seen in mouth breathers who use a nasal mask. These patients may experience increased burping, abdominal bloating or increase in flatulence. Aerophagia is defined by the presence of one symptom during CPAP use. Patients may not complain or may choose to not report these symptoms. It is important for a physician to inquire about these symptoms during clinical encounters. Though there are not definite treatments for this problem, potential treatment options include lowering CPAP pressure, adding expiratory pressure release, or using auto-adjusting CPAP or bi-level PAP. However, none of these treatments are proven to consistently improve symptoms of aerophagia [14].

Interface Challenges

Mask interface plays a very important role in successful treatment of OSA. Mask connects the PAP device via tubing to the patient and delivers the pressure generated by the PAP device to the patient. Selection of suitable mask is very important and at times, can be very challenging to find a suitable mask because of differences in facial features and also constant changes in shape of face, having a beard in male patients and also due to patient's preferences. Sometimes mask will fit well during mask trial session. However while asleep, the muscles of face and jaw relax, causing patient's face to change shape. So the well-fitted mask while awake can become poorly fitted mask during sleep.

Several masks are available in the market such as whole face masks, full face masks, nasal masks, and nasal pillows. Whole face mask extend from forehead to chin of the patient covering eyes, nose, and mouth. Full face masks extend from nasal bridge to chin of the patient covering both nose and mouth. Nasal masks cover just the nose. Nasal pillows snuggly fit into both nostrils.

Overcoming Claustrophobia

Some patients experience claustrophobia when they use the mask. It is more common with full face mask. This could be due to their underlying anxiety as well. This can significantly affect PAP therapy compliance. The best way to overcome this challenge is by desensitization. Prior to PSG titration night or even after that, patients are encouraged to use the mask while awake during the daytime for couple of hours with or without PAP pressure. Once they acclimatize to mask during daytime, they can be encouraged to use it at night time, initially for few hours and gradually increase the time duration of night time use, as the patients get more comfortable. Some patients have a unique challenge of not being able to fall asleep due to anxiety/claustrophobia when they wear the mask, but once they fall asleep they can tolerate the mask well. In such patients using a low dose hypnotic for 1–2 weeks will help them to overcome the anxiety/claustrophobia. Gradually, the dose of hypnotic can be tapered and finally discontinued once patient get used to the mask.

Challenges with the Seal

All masks have a layer of gel/rubber cushion at the point of contact with skin. This cushion will serve multiple purposes. It will provide good seal thus preventing the air leak and also protects the skin from pressure effects of the mask. With the constant use, gel cushion can have wear and tear due to moisture, natural facial oils or friction, resulting in air leak. Also with the change of facial features due to weight changes, beard growth in male can result in poor mask seal. Because of the wear and tear, masks have to be changed, at least in 6 months or earlier as needed.

Mask Air-Leak

The aim of getting a good mask fit is to achieve a stable seal (so that air does not leak out), without compromising patient's comfort. Air leak up to 50 ml/min is considered acceptable. Ill-fitted masks can result in significant air leak. Significant PAP mask leak may exceed patient's PAP ability to maintain the prescribed pressure, may impair the machine's sensors ability to detect what's going on, and may thereby prevent PAP's algorithms from properly responding to ongoing respiratory events. Thus, OSA is usually undertreated due to significant mask leak. So the leak problem has to be addressed as soon as possible. Depending on the site of leak, air can blow into the eyes as well; resulting dryness of cornea, which can be very uncomfortable to the patient due to burning sensation in the eyes.

Mouth Air-Leak

Mouth leak happens if patient sleeps with mouth open and air leaks out of patient's mouth during therapy. This is mainly seen in patients who use nasal mask. Opening mouth during sleep can either be out of habit, or could be due to a blocked nose. Mouth leak can be very uncomfortable and leave patient with a dry mouth. (It is also very noisy; if it doesn't wake patient, it might wake the bed partner.) If it happens every now and then, patient might be able to stop it by wearing a chin strap to keep his/her mouth closed, or by using a humidifier to stop nose getting blocked. If mouth leak happens a lot, patient may need to use a full face mask, which covers both patient's nose and mouth, so even if patient breathe through his/her mouth while asleep, air will not leak out.

Mask Pressure

Mask is connected to the face via headgear. This headgear will keep the mask in position. If the mask is applied very tight, it can cause significant pressure at the point of contact to the skin. The most common side effect of using mask is skin rash at the point of contact. However in some patients it can cause significant skin irritation, abrasion, or even skin break down. Patients think that applying mask very tightly will prevent mask leak. It is not at all true. Excessively tightening of mask can actually worsen the leak. One has to use just right amount of pressure that is needed to hold the mask in place avoiding air leak. Also mask leaks can cause significant air blowing sound. Several patients, especially their bed partners have complained about this noise waking them from sleep, thus causing sleep disruption.

In summary, air leak can be due to mask leak, mouth leak, and due to not using right about of pressure to hold the mask in correct position. This problem poses significant challenges in terms of delivering adequate PAP to the patient, causing discomfort to the patient and to the bed partner, which in turn can affect the compliance. So patients can try few different things to overcome this challenge.

Patient who have mouth leak and who do not want to use chin strap can use whole face mask. These masks cover almost entire face, some patients like complete face masks over using chin straps for mouth leaks.

Mask liners are specially designed mask accessories that prevent the silicone gel of PAP masks from coming into direct contact with the face during PAP therapy. They are made from natural fibers that absorb oils and moisture. They are flexible enough to adjust to the inherent contours of the face. They can also be used to reduce air leaks that cause sleep disturbances. There mask liners are commercially available. A patient can also craft them at home. Patient has to take a soft cloth and cut it to the size of mask. Patient has to place the mask liner first on the face and then place the mask on the mask liner. So mask rests on the mask liner, and liners absorb the moisture, natural facial oils, and also prevent air leak.

Alternatively, commercially available PAP gel may be the answer for mask leak and skin irritation. PAP gel creates a thin, smooth, adaptable seal around PAP mask cushion that stops air from escaping, eliminates distracting noises, and improves overall therapy and leak levels. PAP gel also helps to restore dry skin while it reduces irritation from mask cushion. PAP gel's adaptable seal allows many users to loosen their mask headgear without compromising the mask seal for improved comfort and therapy success.

Despite trying several masks, some patients may not find the right mask for them. Being patient is the most important thing while choosing the right mask that is suitable for a patient. Also, it is very important to master the technique of wearing a mask. Patient has to pay close attention during mask trail session and learn the proper technique from technician.

PAP Device Challenges

PAP device delivers positive pressure. Over the course of years, the size and weight of the PAP devices have considerably decreased making it easy for the patient. The available compact machines help the patient to move the machine easily from one place to another inside their homes and also carry with her/him during travel. However, there are few challenges that a patient may face while using the PAP machine.

Malfunctioning Device

Noise Level

Compared to the older machines, newer machines generate significantly less noise. However, some patients or their bed partners may be very sensitive to noise of any kind. This can disturb their sleep leading to a failure of the primary purpose of using PAP therapy. Such patients or their bed partners should be advised to try using ear plugs if they prove helpful. However, many patients eventually get used to the small noise that is emitted from the machine over the course of time.

Also different levels of noise are generated depending on the type of PAP machines. Bi-level-PAP machines generate more noise than continuous PAP machines due to a change in the pressure with every breath. Auto PAP machines also have similar issues as the pressure changes to meet the patient's requirements. Even with such variability, the noise generated by these machines is generally minimal.

Another important aspect a patient needs to remember is to check air filters from time to time, as the clogged air filters can contribute to a higher level of noise. Air filters need to be changed routinely, i.e., on a monthly basis or sooner if there is any change in the color or if the noise from the machine is increasing. Despite these remedial actions, if the patient finds that the machine continues to make noise that is not tolerated by the patient or the bed partner, it is advisable to speak with the machine supplier to see if there are any other problems with this machine.

Tubing Problem

PAP machine are connected to the mask via tubing. Through this tube, the pressure is delivered to the mask. Some people experience challenges with the tubing. The standard tube is 6 ft long. Some patients find the tubing limiting their movement in the bed, especially from a side to side position. During sleep, sudden movement of the patient may cause the tube to get disconnected either from the mask or from the device and as a result of the high pressure air flow, an accompanying loud noise is typically generated, which wakes up the patient and their bed partner resulting in unwarranted sleep disturbances. A few solutions are available for this problem. The first solution is placing the PAP device behind patient's head near the top of her/his pillow, or position behind the headboard/bed post. Most PAP suppliers offer an inexpensive tubing "lift" to help with tube positioning for better sleep. They are generally easy to use, and the lift's small frame is held in place between the box spring and mattress. The lift holds the tubing above the head allowing for better freedom of movement. Some companies supply tubes up to 10 ft. long as well. So using longer tubing such as 10 ft. tubing will give more room for patient to turn around.

Humidification Problems

One of the important challenges a patient may face while using PAP therapy is dryness of the upper airway. Some patients complain of some dryness, which they find it manageable. However, other patients experience severe dryness of the upper airway, which can potentially lead to poor PAP therapy compliance. Noncompliance is an issue in about 10% of patients due to dryness and irritation of the mucosal lining of the respiratory tract [15]. Rarely, patients also complain of nose bleeds because of severe upper airway dryness. In order to improve patient's comfort and to improve the compliance every PAP device is equipped with a humidifier and the patient can self-adjust the degree of humidification to best meet her/his needs. These heated humidifiers are used to increase humidity and decrease the dryness and thus may help mitigate such noncompliance.

Few important simple steps need to be taken by the patient on a daily basis while using humidification. PAP devices are equipped with humidifier chambers and only distilled water should be used for humidification, as the use of regular tap water can result in deposition of minerals on the walls of tubing system and thus potentially damage the tubing. Distilled water is inexpensive and generally available in pharmacies. Some patients may require higher settings of humidification, and this may result in the usage of distilled water within the PAP machine at a faster pace, thus requiring refilling every night, or even twice a night. Air leaks from the mask can also result in loss of humidification, which may also result in requiring frequent refilling. So if patient has to re-fill humidifier chamber nightly or even twice nightly, it is important to check for mask/mouth air leak and if present, then have to take necessary steps to rectify the problem. At the same time, patient should make sure that left over water in the chamber should not be allowed to sit for long periods of time as it can result in microbial infestation and increases chances of respiratory infections.

Despite using humidification, if the patient experiences dryness, simple measures can be undertaken to improve the symptoms. Mild mouth/throat dryness can be alleviated with just drinking some water. Some patients benefit from using saline mouth and nasal sprays, Biotene mouth washes, gels, and sprays which are widely available over the counter. Patients who used these have reported that they experienced improvement in their symptoms.

Condensation of humidity in tubing and in the mask is another concern. When the humidity from the humidifier enters an unheated tube, the difference in temperature may cause condensation to occur. The warmer the humidifier air and the colder the tubing, the more condensation occur. Patients may experience condensed water running into their nose or mouth, which can wake them up from sleep. This can be avoided by simply placing the PAP device below the level of patient, so that condensed water will be collected, back in the humidifier chamber. Most suppliers offer inexpensive insulating hose covers, which help avoid this problem. Heated tubing is available which can keep the temperature of the tubing above the room temperature, and this will prevent the condensation formation in the tubing. A heated tube delivers the warm, moist air from the heated humidifier to the PAP mask. Thus using heated tubes will maximize the benefit of the humidifier.

Patients using heated humidifiers without regard to good hygienic practices in maintaining their humidifiers by thorough cleansing and replacing their breathing tubes showed a dramatic increase in upper airway infections, compared with those who cared for their equipment regularly, when examined over a 6-month interval (52.4% vs. 13.3%; $p < 0.05$) [16]. It is thus important to educate patients on the risks of not appropriately maintaining their humidifiers and related equipment. It is important to advise patients to empty leftover water, rinse chamber, and let it air-dry every morning. To remove any possible bacterial film and related contamination, the chamber will need to be soaked for an hour with a solution that is one part white distilled vinegar and two parts tap water. The chamber would then need to be rinsed with clear tap water and air dried. Based on the manufacturer, some humidifier chambers are dish washer safe as well.

Contour PAP Pillows

There are several accessories available in market, which claims to increase the comfort of the patient while using PAP therapy and thus increase the compliance. One of them is contour PAP pillows. These contour PAP pillow claims to improve sleep comfort for all PAP users, PAP compliance, neck support, spine alignment, and airway alignment. They also claim to reduce mask leaks, pressure on mask and face, and mask discomfort. These may help with individual patients, but no controlled studies are available to support this information.

Device Maintenance

Just like any other equipment, PAP devices need regular servicing. Patients need to carry their devices to the DME (durable medical equipment) provider in a timely manner. Most of the time, local DME providers do a fantastic job in offering this service. They check for mask leaks, tubing leaks, humidification chamber leaks, and humidification function and also make sure that patient is on correct prescribed settings. During these sessions, they offer one on one brief education classes, which can help the patients a lot in the long run. So patients have to make an attempt to meet with their DME providers on a regular basis.

Travel

With the advances in technology, battery-powered PAP machines are now available. Once travel is planned, the patient should contact his supplier for battery-powered PAP devices. This will help the patient to travel anywhere, including camping. Further, airport staffs are generally well aware of PAP devices and this makes travel more convenient with a PAP device.

Follow-Up

Treatment Compliance

As usage increase more than 4 h per night, subjective sleepiness, then objective sleepiness, lastly, quality of life measures improve [3]. A 5-year cumulative survival highest in group of CPAP therapy greater than 6 h per night compared to group with 1–6 h per night and less than 1 h per night. More than 5 h per night CPAP use had a drop in mean arterial BP of about 4 mmHg [17]. A higher percentage of patients achieved normal functioning with longer duration nightly CPAP nightly CPAP therapy [18].

With advances in the technology, these devices can measures patient's PAP therapy compliance, number of hours of PAP therapy usage, average leak, and residual AHI. Some machines have SD card which can be removed from the device and patients can carry to the DME provider who will download the data for review. Now with further advancement in technology, DME providers can remotely access the PAP compliance data and give it to patients or send to their health care providers for review. It is very important to review this data in a timely fashion as this will give an estimate of patient's compliance and treatment effectiveness. It is also important to document it in the patient's clinic notes for insurance purposes.

Persistent Symptoms

The main purpose of PAP therapy is to keep the upper airway open, so that patient can breathe comfortably and continuously without any interruption and thus avoid excessive daytime sleepiness. Despite the optimal compliance with PAP therapy, some patient may have frequent awakenings from sleep and may have non-restorative sleep in the morning and may continue to experience excessive daytime sleepiness problem. There is a possibility of patients perceiving these persistent symptoms as treatment failure, resulting in giving up on the PAP therapy. Actually in such situations, other etiologies need to be considered, as patient may have more than one diagnoses. For example, along with sleep apnea, patients may have narcolepsy or some patients may just have residual daytime sleepiness despite optimal treatment compliance. These patients may need further investigations and additional treatments. So it is always important to have regular follow-up with sleep medicine physician or at least with primary care physician.

Alternative Therapies

Some patients after starting on PAP therapy, for several reasons may not like the therapy and may discontinue the treatment. In such patients, every attempt should be made to understand the problem and try to solve it. Despite several interventions and counseling sessions, if patient is not willing to try PAP therapy, then alternative treatment options should be discussed. Depending on the type of sleep apnea, underlying precipitating factors should be treated or current treatment should be optimized. For mild sleep apnea, oral appliance devices, positional therapy with positional therapy device can be tried. And in severe cases, combination of therapies like oral appliance devices and positional therapy or even surgical interventions like uvulo-palato-pharyngeoplasty, mandibular advancement surgeries, etc. can be considered.

Key Points

1. For patients who cannot fall asleep due to high PAP pressures, starting PAP therapy at a lower pressure setting and ramping up to target pressure over a period of 30–45 min will help the patient fall asleep.

2. Exhalation relief setting is a feature in which the pressure delivered by the machine will automatically be lowered during exhalation period, depending on the settings chosen.
3. In approximately 56–75% of patients with obstructive sleep apnea (OSA), the frequency and duration of apneas are influenced by body position. This is referred to as position-dependent OSA or POSA.
4. In patients with intolerance of higher pressure settings, apnea during supine sleep can be alleviated with positional therapy with avoidance of supine sleep with positional therapy device and apnea in side sleep can be alleviated with low PAP pressure.
5. Another form of positional therapy is elevation of head end of the bed (HOB). Elevating head of the bed itself can result in decreased collapsibility of upper air ways collapsibility. Elevating HOB just by 30–45° itself will decrease severity of sleep apnea by 25–30%.
6. Techniques that can be tried to address aerophagia with PAP therapy include lowering CPAP pressure, adding expiratory pressure release, or using auto-adjusting CPAP or bi-level PAP.
7. Mask liners are specially designed mask accessories that prevent the silicone gel of PAP masks from coming into direct contact with the face during PAP therapy.

References

1. Kapur V, Strohl KP, Redline S, Iber C, O'Connor G, Nieto J. Underdiagnosis of sleep apnea syndrome in U.S. communities. Sleep Breath. 2002;6:49–54.
2. Weaver T, Grunstein R. Adherence to continuous positive airway pressure therapy. Proc Am Thorac Soc. 2008;5:173–8.
3. Weaver T, et al. Relationship between hours of CPAP use and achieving normal levels of sleepiness and daily functioning. Sleep. 2007;30(6):711–9.
4. Weaver T, Sawyer A. Adherence to continuous positive airway pressure treatment for obstructive sleep apnea: implications for future interventions. Indian J Med Res. 2010;131:248–58.
5. Somers VK, White DP, Amin R, Abraham WT, Costa F, Culebras A, Daniels S, Floras JS, Hunt CE, Olson LJ, Pickering TG, Russell R, Woo M, Young T. Sleep apnea and cardiovascular disease. Circulation. 2008;118(10):1080–111.
6. Young T, Peppard P, Gottlieb D. Epidemiology of obstructive sleep apnea. Am J Respir Crit Care Med. 2002;165:1217–39.
7. Siccoli M, Pepperell J, Kohler M, Craig S, Davies R, Stradling J. Effects of continuous positive airway pressure on quality of life in patients with moderate to severe obstructive sleep apnea: data from a randomized control trial. Sleep. 2008;31(11):1551–8.
8. Rodenstein D. Sleep apnea: traffic and occupational accidents-individual risks, socioeconomic and legal implications. Respiration. 2009;78:241–8.
9. Wittmann V, Rodenstein D. Health care costs and sleep apnea syndrome. Sleep Med Rev. 2004;8(4):269–79.
10. Boyaci H, Garcar K, Baris SA, Basygit I, Yildiz F. Positive airway pressure device compliance of patient with obstructive sleep apnea syndrome. Adv Clin Exp Med. 2013;22(6):809–15.
11. Sanna A. Obstructive sleep apnoea, motor vehicle accidents, and work performance. Chron Respir Dis. 2013;10(1):29–33.

12. Ravesloot MJ, White D, Heinzer R, Oksenberg A, Pépin JL. Efficacy of the new generation of devices for positional therapy for patients with positional obstructive sleep apnea: a systematic review of the literature and meta-analysis. J Clin Sleep Med. 2017;13(6):813–24.
13. Neill AM, Angus SM, Sajkov D, McEvoy RD. Effects of sleep posture on upper airway stability in patients with obstructive sleep apnea. Am J Respir Crit Care Med. 1997;155(1):199–204.
14. Harding SM. CPAP-related aerophagia: awareness first. J Clin Sleep Med. 2013;9(1):19–20.
15. Mador MJ, Krauza M, Pervez A, Pierce D, Braun M. Effect of heated humidification on compliance and quality of life in patients with sleep apnea using nasal continuous positive airway pressure. Chest. 2005;128:2151–8.
16. Sanner BM, Fluerenbrock N, Kleiber-Imbeck A, Mueller JB, Zidek W. Effect of continuous positive airway pressure therapy on infectious complications in patients with obstructive sleep apnea syndrome. Respiration. 2001;68:483–7.
17. Campos-Rodriguez F, et al. Mortality in obstructive sleep apnea-hypopnea patients treated with positive airway pressure. Chest. 2005;128(2):624–33.
18. Antic NA, Catcheside P, Buchan C, et al. The effect of CPAP in normalizing daytime sleepiness, quality of life and neurocognitive function in patients with moderate to severe OSA. Sleep. 2011;34(1):111–9.

Appendix

Table A.1 Segmental innervation of the spinal cord

Spinal cord segment	Major muscles innervated	Muscle action	Deep tendon reflexes
C1, C2	Rectus lateralis, rectus capitis anterior, longus capitis, longus cervicis, sternocleidomastoid	Neck flexion	
C3	Longus capitis, longus cervicis, trapezius	Neck lateral flexion	
C4	Diaphragm, trapezius, levator scapularis, scalenus anterior and medius	Shoulder elevation	
C5	Deltoid, supraspinatus, infraspinatus, teres minor, biceps, scalenus anterior and medius	Shoulder abduction	Bicep reflex
C6	Serratus anterior, subscapularis, teres major, latissimus dorsi, pectoralis major, biceps, brachialis, brachioradialis, extensor carpi radialis longus, supinator, scalenus anterior, medius, and posterior	Elbow flexion and wrist extension	Brachioradialis reflex
C7	Serratus anterior, latissimus dorsi, pectoralis major and minor, triceps, pronator teres, extensor carpi radialis longus, flexor digitorum superficialis, flexor carpi radialis. Extensor carpi radialis brevis, extensor digitorum, extensor digiti minimi	Elbow extension and wrist flexion	Triceps reflex
C8	Pectoralis major and minor, triceps, flexor digitorum superficialis, flexor digitorum profundus, flexor pollicis longus, pronator quadratus, flexor carpi, abductor pollicis longus, extensor pollicis longus, extensor pollicis brevis, extensor indicis, abductor pollicis brevis, flexor pollicis brevis, opponens pollicis	Thumb extension	
T1	Flexor digitorum profundus, intrinsic muscles of hand, flexor pollicis brevis, ppponens pollicis	Finger abduction and adduction	
L1, L2	Psoas, Iliacus, sartorius, gracilis, pectineus, adductor longus, adductor brevis	Hip flexion	
L3	Quadriceps, adductor longus, magnus, and brevis	Knee flexion	Patellar tendon reflex

© Springer International Publishing AG, part of Springer Nature 2018
R. Govindarajan, P. C. Bollu (eds.), *Sleep Issues in Neuromuscular Disorders*,
https://doi.org/10.1007/978-3-319-73068-4

Spinal cord segment	Major muscles innervated	Muscle action	Deep tendon reflexes
L4	Tibialis, quadriceps, tensor fascia lata, adductor magnus, obturator externus, tibialis posterior	Ankle dorsiflexion	Patellar tendon reflex
L5	Extensor hallucis longus, extensor digitorum longus, gluteus medius and minimus, obturator internus, semimembranosus, popliteus	Toe extension	Tibialis posterior reflex
S1	Gastrocnemius, soleus, gluteus maximus, obturator internus, piriformis, biceps femoris, semitendinosus, popliteus, peroneus longus and brevis, extensor digitorum brevis	Ankle plantar flexion	Achilles reflex
S2	Biceps femoris, gastrocnemius, soleus, piriformis, flexor digitorum longus, flexor hallucis longus, intrinsic muscles of foot	Knee flexion	
S3	Intrinsic muscles of foot, flexor hallucis brevis, flexor digitorum brevis, extensor digitorum brevis	Rectal sphincter tone	

Table A.2 Anatomical localization and causes of lower motor neuron lesions

Localization	Causes	Signs and symptoms
Spinal cord		
Foramen magnum	Meningioma, chordoma, atlanto-axial subluxation	Spastic quadriparesis, neck pain and stiffness, facial numbness, ipsilateral Horner Syndrome
Anterior cord	Anterior spinal artery infarction	Upper and lower motor paralysis, spinothalamic sensory loss, sphincter dysfunction
Central cord	Syringomyelia	Paraparesis, wasting and fasciculations in arms, sensory loss in shawl distribution
Posterior cord	Extrinsic compression, vitamin B-12 deficiency, multiple sclerosis	Loss of proprioception and vibration, sensation of constricting bands, tingling, numbness
Conus medullaris	Intrinsic tumors, extrinsic compression	Lower sacral saddle sensory loss, sphincter disturbance, lower back and perineal pain, foot and ankle weakness
Cauda equina	Extrinsic compression, spinal stenosis	Early sphincter dysfunction, paraparesis, sensory loss and weakness in multiple bilateral dermatomes
Anterior horn	Amyotrophic lateral sclerosis (ALS), poliomyelitis	Progressive flaccid weakness, wasting, fasciculations
Nerve root/ plexus	Mechanical injury, malignancy, external compression	Single limb, and/or radicular weakness, pain and paresthesias with indistinctly demarcated sensory loss, absent deep tendon reflexes, no muscular atrophy or fasciculations
Peripheral nerve	Guillain–Barré syndrome (GBS), chronic inflammatory demyelinating polyneuropathy	Focal or distal severe weakness, prominent muscle atrophy, hyporeflexia, and fasciculations. Sharply demarcated sensory loss, pain and paresthesias in nerve distribution, and autonomic disturbances
Neuromuscular junction	Myasthenia gravis, Lambert–Eaton syndrome, botulism	Fluctuating weakness, diplopia

Table A.3 Classification of deep tendon reflexes

Reflexes	Associated muscle group	Associated spinal dermatomal	Associated spinal nerve root	Site of stimulus for reflex	Conditions with abnormal reflexes
Biceps	Bicep brachii	C5	Musculo cutaneous nerve	Bicep brachii tendon at cubital fossa	Myopathy neuropathy, poliomyelitis, neuritis, hyperthyroidism
Brachioradialis	Extensor carpi radialis	C6	Radial nerve	Brachioradialis tendon at radial styloid process in wrist	Myopathy neuropathy, poliomyelitis, neuritis, hyperthyroidism
Triceps	Tricep brachii	C7	Radial nerve	Tricep tendon at back of elbow joint	Myopathy neuropathy, poliomyelitis, neuritis, hyperthyroidism
Patellar	Tibialis anterior, quadriceps	L4	Femoral nerve	Patellar tendon below the patella	Lumbar radiculopathy
Babinski	Extensor hallucis longus	L4-5, S1-2	Tibial nerve	Lateral side of sole of foot	Disc herniation, lumbar radiculopathy
Achilles	Gastrocnemius, soleus	S1	Tibial nerve	Achilles tendon in a dorsiflexed foot	Disc herniation, hypothyroidism, diabetes, neurosyphilis, alcoholism

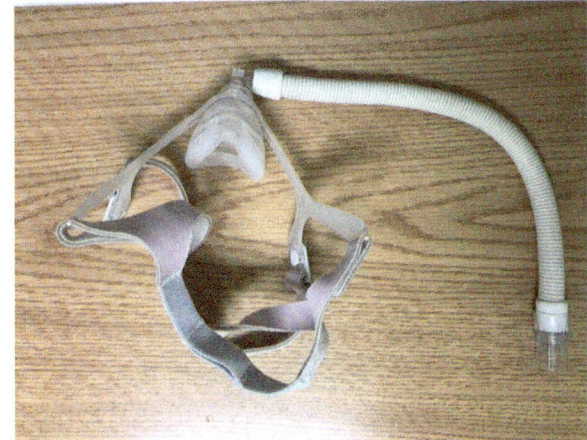

Fig. A.1 PAP headgear along with a nasal mask. The elastic material of the headgear helps hold the mask in place and gives a good seal. The headgear comes in different sizes and shapes depending on the model. After a few months of usage, the headgear is usually replaced due to the wear and tear and loss of elasticity

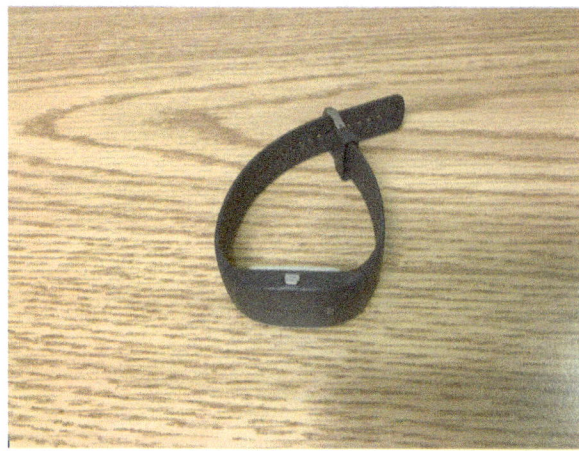

Fig. A.2 Actigraphy watch: This is worn on the wrist and helps to track the body movements and inactivity. Actigraphy recording is usually done for 2–4 weeks to monitor the sleep–wake patterns of patients. The inactivity recorded in the actigraphy watch is used as a surrogate for sleep in analyzing the sleep–wake rhythms. Patients are encouraged to wear the equipment day and night as much as possible. Sometimes, patients are asked to record their sleep–wake rhythms on a separate diary while performing actigraphy recording

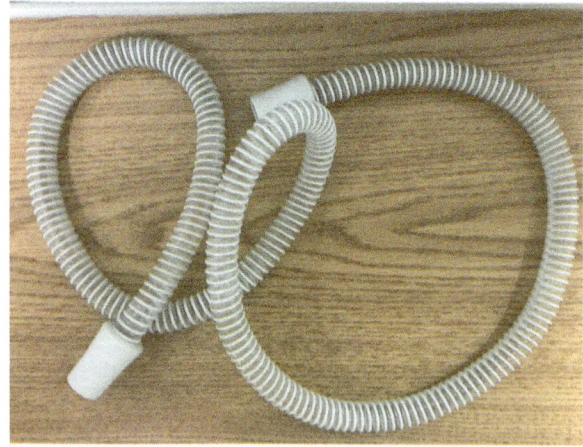

Fig. A.3 Tubing: Tubing connects the headgear to the PAP device and helps deliver the pressure generated at the PAP machine to the interface. The tubing shown below is quite simple and consists of a plastic hollow tube and a surrounding molded plastic with rubber rubber ends. Some modern tubing comes with a heating coil that helps prevent condensation of the humidity inside the tubing

Appendix 157

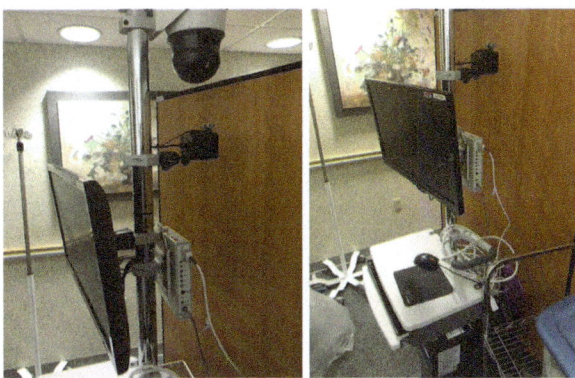

Fig. A.4 Portable monitor: This portable PSG equipment has audio and video recording along with EEG monitoring but may not have all the other channels that a conventional PSG recording equipment has. This equipment is typically used to obtain PSGs on patients that are admitted to the hospital who can't obtain regular PSGs. The equipment is brought to the patient's room and set up

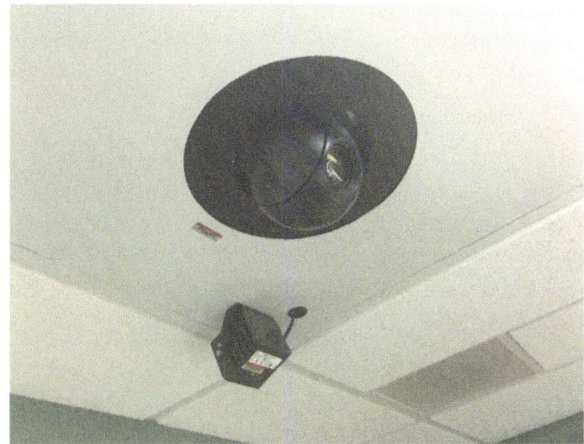

Fig. A.5 Video recording of PSG: Video cameras (regular and night vision cameras) mounted on the ceiling (typically) will record the video during the PSG

Fig. A.6 Audio recording: The microphone above the patient's head (white device—in this picture) will record audio

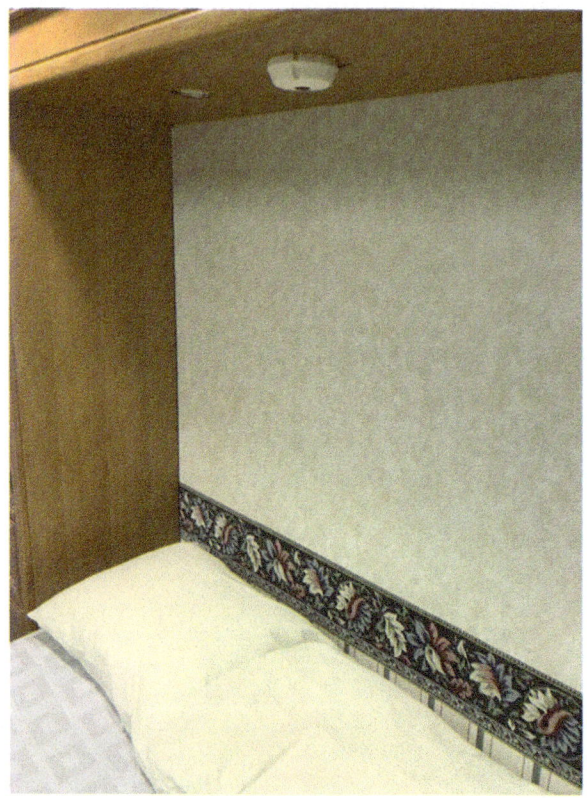

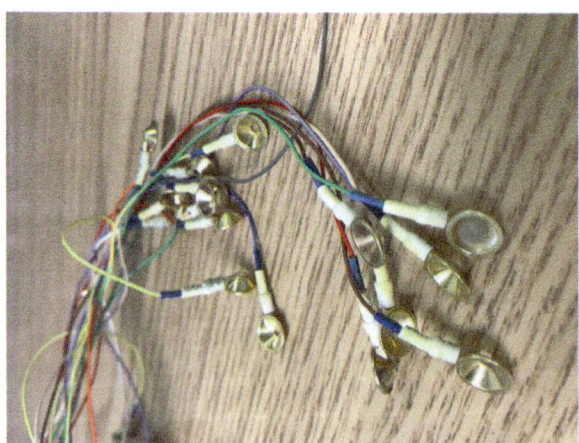

Fig. A.7 Wiring and electrodes

Fig. A.8 Home sleep study recording: The equipment is given or mailed to the patient along with the instructions to set it up

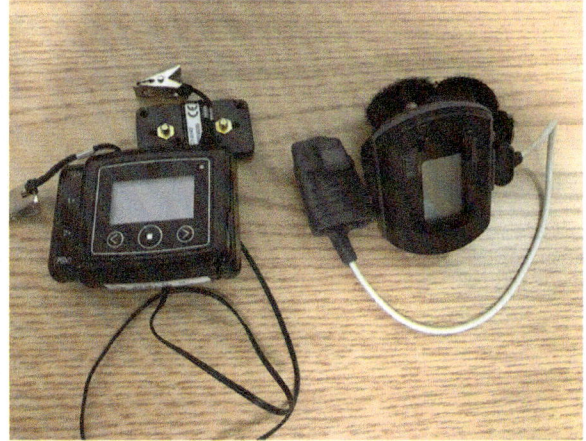

Fig. A.9 Headbox: This acts as an interface into which all the wiring from the recording electrodes go in. It is connected to the computer for data acquisition

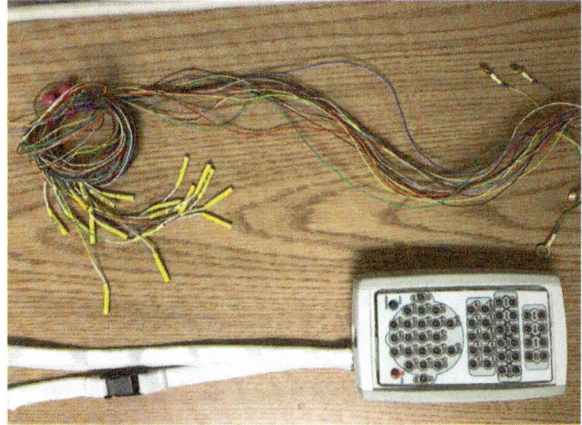

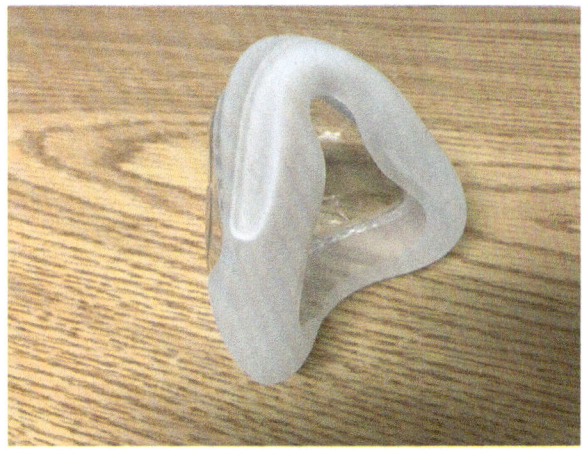

Fig. A.10 A nasal mask interface. The soft silicone helps with the seal all along the area of contact and minimizes the air leak

Fig. A.11 Skin prep gel used to clean the skin. Conductive electrode paste that is applied to the electrodes before setting them up on the scalp

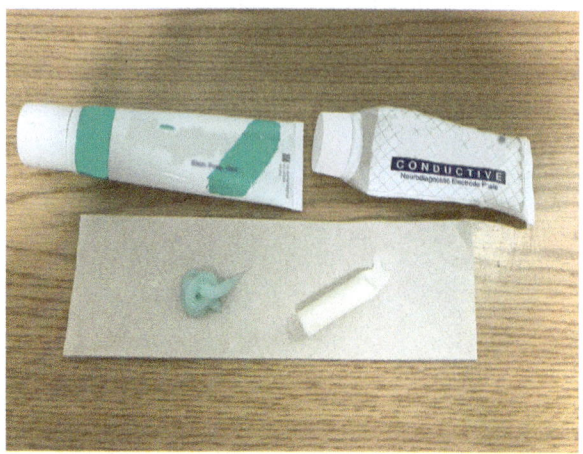

Fig. A.12 Chest and abdominal belts that record thoraco-abdominal excursions during the PSG

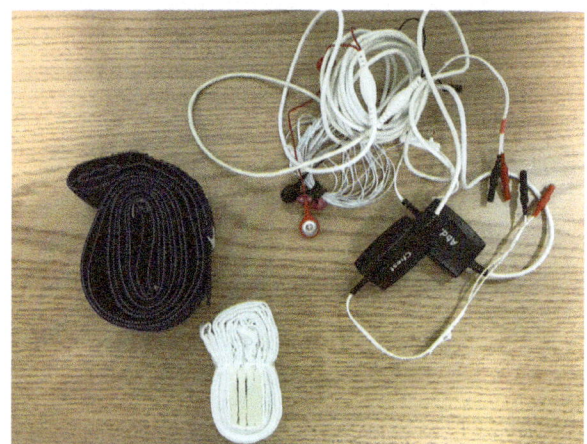

Sample CPAP Titration Protocol

> Start with a CPAP pressure of 4 cm

If
- 2 or more obstructive apneas
- 3 or more Hypopneas
- 5 or more RERAs
- Greater than 3 min of loud snoring

> Increase CPAP pressure by 1 cm of H_2O

If
- 2 or more obstructive apneas
- 3 or more Hypopneas
- 5 or more RERAs
- Greater than 3 min of loud snoring

> Increase CPAP pressure by 1 cm of H_2O till 30 min or more sleep without respiratory events is noted

Further exploration of PAP pressure can be considered after no clear respiratory events are noted.

At 15 cm of CPAP pressure, BiPAP can be considered for continued respiratory events.

Maximum CPAP pressure is 20 cm of H_2O.

Fig. A.13 Neuromuscular junction

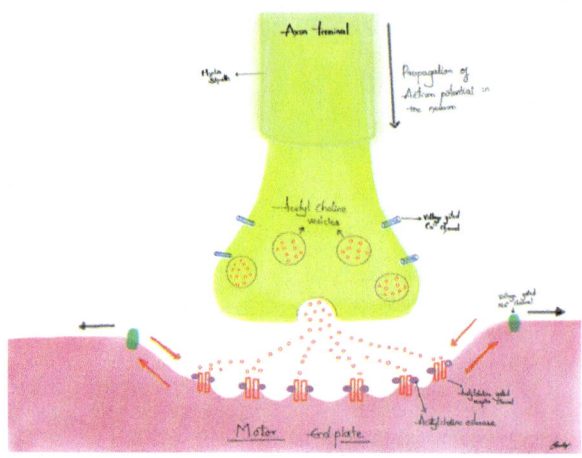

Fig. A.14 Dermatomes of upper limb

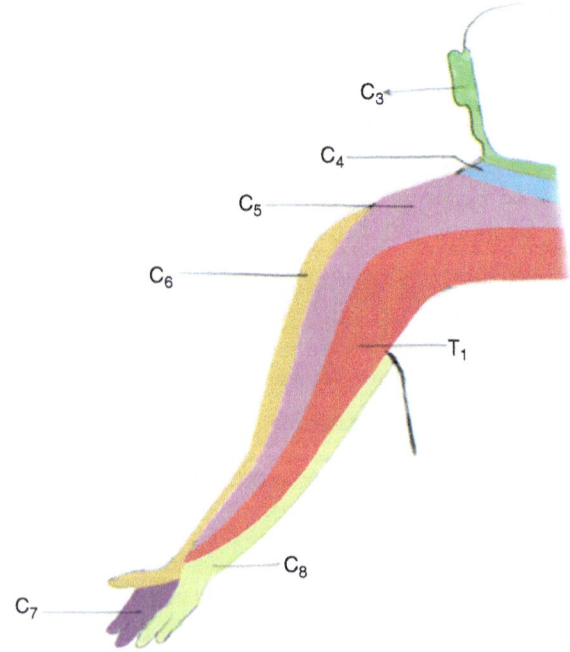

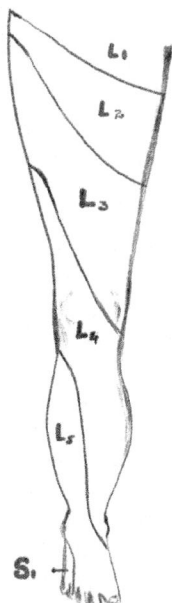

Fig. A.15 Dermatomes of lower limb

Index

A
AASM Manual for the Scoring of Sleep and Associated Events, 2
Acid maltase deficiency, 64
Actigraphy, 16, 17
Adult nonobese diabetics, 98
Aerophagia, 142
Air swallowing, 142
American Academy of Sleep Medicine (AASM), 2, 10, 16, 17, 19, 104, 105
Amyotrophic lateral sclerosis (ALS)
   bulbar onset, 47
   diagnosis, 47
   frontotemporal dementia, 47, 48
   incidence, 46
   limb/spinal onset, 47
   monomelic, 48
Apnea-hypopnea index, 96
Arterial oxygen content (PaO_2), 9, 29, 130
Arterial oxygen saturation (SaO_2), 9, 11–13
Average volume assured pressure support (AVAPS), 124

B
Becker's muscular dystrophy, 64
Benign epileptiform transients of sleep (BETS), 6, 7
Bi-level positive airway pressure (BIPAP), 36, 37, 109, 124, 133
Botulism
   clinical diagnosis, 85
   clinical features, 85
   laboratory and electrodiagnostic testing, 86
   treatment, 86
   types, 85
Botzinger complex, 25
Breathing control, 25, 26

C
Capillary endothelial cell hyperplasia, 97
Capnography, 9, 53
Charcot–Marie–Tooth (CMT) patients, 95
Circadian rhythm disorders, 67, 68
Claustrophobia, 143
Common mode rejection ratio (CMRR), 3
Continuous positive airway pressure (CPAP), 3, 9, 15, 16, 18, 90, 96, 109, 121, 123, 124, 133, 139, 141, 142, 148, 149, 161
Contour PAP pillows, 148

D
Daily sleep interference scale (DSIS), 95
Daytime nap polysomnography (DPSG), 106
Diabetic neuropathy (DPN), 98
Diaphragm pacing, 55
Diaphragm palsy, 96
Diurnal tests, 105, 106
Dorsal respiratory group (DRG), 25
Duchenne muscular dystrophy (DMD), 62, 64–66, 108, 111

E
Electrocardiography (EKG), 3, 6, 8, 11–16, 18, 84
Electroencephalography (EEG)
   abnormal pattern, 5, 6
   epileptiform-like patterns, 7
   Jack box, 5
   mimickers, 6
   normal pattern, 5
   procedure, 5
   sharp artifacts, 6
   sharp transients

Electroencephalography (EEG) (cont.)
   BETS/SSS, 7
   hypnogogic hypersynchrony, 7
   K-complex, 6
   Mu rhythm, 6
   posterior slow waves of youth, 7
   POSTS, 6
   vertex sharp waves, 7
   wicket rhythms, 7
Electromyography (EMG), 7, 8
Electrooculography (EOG), 2–4, 8, 15–17
Emery-Dreifuss muscular dystrophy, 64
End-tidal CO_2 monitoring, 15
Epworth sleepiness scale (ESS) scoring, 87–89, 106
Erasmus GBS respiratory insufficiency score (EGRIS), 32, 33
Excessive daytime sleepiness (EDS), 16, 66, 67, 87, 88
Excitatory postsynaptic potentials (EPSP), 5
Expiratory positive airway pressure, 123

F
Fascioscapulohumeral muscular dystrophy (FSHD), 64, 65
Finger pulse oximetry, 9, 17
First-generation ventilators, 119
Forced vital capacity (FVC), 28, 29, 31, 32, 35, 53, 55, 96, 133, 135
Forehead reflectance oximetry, 17
Fourth-generation ventilators, 120

G
Guillain-Barré syndrome, 23, 27, 31, 32, 34–36, 133, 135, 136

H
Hereditary sensory motor neuropathy, 96
High-frequency filter, 3
High-pass filter, see Low-frequency filter
Hirayama disease, 48
Home mechanical ventilation (HMV), 111
Home sleep testing (HST), 17, 159
Home ventilation strategies, 134
Hypercapnia, 28, 29, 37, 64, 65, 90, 102, 118, 122, 133, 135
Hypersomnia, 66
Hypnogogic hypersynchrony, 7

I
Inhibitory postsynaptic potentials (IPSP), 5
Insomnia
   motor neuron disorder, 52
   myopathies and muscular dystrophies, 64, 65
Inspiratory positive airway pressure, 122
Insufficient sleep syndrome, 66
International Classification of Sleep Disorders (ICSD-3), 62, 64–67, 104
International Ten-Twenty System, 4
Internuclear ophthalmoplegia (INO), 77
Invasive mechanical ventilation, 109–110

J
Jack box, 5

K
K-complex, 6
Kennedy's disease, 46
Kleine-Levin syndrome, 66

L
Lambert–Eaton myasthenic syndrome (LEMS)
   causes, 82
   course of, 82, 83
   definition, 82
   diagnosis, 83, 84
   epidemiology, 82
   signs and symptoms, 83
   sleep issues, 89
   treatment
      cholinesterase inhibitors, 84
      immunotherapy, 84
      tumor therapy, 84
Laser-assisted uvulopalatopharyngoplasty (LAUP), 10, 19
Late Onset Spinal Motor Neuronopathy (LOSMoN), 46
Limb-Girdle muscular dystrophy (LGMD), 64, 103, 113
Low-frequency filter, 3
Low-pass filter, see High-frequency filter

M
Maintenance of wakefulness test (MWT), 16
Maximal expiratory pressure (MEP), 28, 29, 31, 32, 34–39
Maximal inspiratory pressure (MIP), 28, 29, 31, 32, 34, 36–39, 135

Index

Mechanical ventilation (MV)
  CPAP, 121
  in GBS, 31–33
    algorithm, 33, 35
    cardiovascular autonomic
      dysfunction, 33
    EGRIS, 32
    endotracheal MV, 32
    motor weakness, 33
    MRC sum score, 32
    prolonged intubation, 35, 36
    respiratory failure risk, 32
    risk factors, 33, 34
  myasthenia gravis, 36–38
  peak pressure, 122
  PEEP, 121
  plateau pressure, 122
  tidal volume and minute ventilation, 122
Medical Research Council (MRC)
  sum score, 32–34
Montage
  CPAP trial, 12
  intrathoracic pressure monitoring, 12
  multiple sleep latency test, 15
  REM sleep behavior disorder, 14
  seizures/suspected parasomnias, 13
  standard polysomnogram, 11
Motor neuron disorders
  ALS
    bulbar onset, 47
    diagnosis, 47
    frontotemporal dementia, 47, 48
    incidence, 46
    limb/spinal onset, 47
    monomelic, 48
    chemo-sensitivity and respiratory
      control, 50
    definition, 44
    diaphragm weakness, 50, 51
    PLS, 48
    PMA, 48
    SDB (see Sleep disordered breathing
      (SDB))
    sleep diagnosis
      nocturnal pulse oximetry, 53
      PSG, 53
      pulmonary function testing, 53
      sleep history and clinical
        examination, 52, 53
      SNIP, 54
    sleep disorders
      insomnia, 52
      PLMS, 52
      RLS, 52
    sleep fragmentation, 51
    sleep history and clinical examination, 53
    sleep management
      comorbid conditions, 54
      diaphragm pacing, 55
      insomnia, 54
      NIV, 55
      RLS, 54
      sleep hygiene, 54
      tracheostomy, 55
    sleep stages and respiration, 50
  SMA
    clinical features, 44
    incidence, 44
    LOSMoN, 46
    SMA-LED, 46
    SPSMA, 46
    type 0, 45
    type 1, 45
    type 2, 45
    type 3, 45
    type 4, 45
  spinal and bulbar muscular
    atrophy (X-linked), 46
  upper airway resistance, 50
Mu rhythm, 6
Multifocal motor neuropathy with
  conduction block (MMNCB),
  96, 97
Multiple sleep latency test (MSLT), 8, 16, 90
Muscle-specific tyrosine kinase (MuSK), 75,
  76, 78, 79
Muscular dystrophies, see Myopathies and
  muscular dystrophies
Myasthenia gravis (MG)
  causes, 76
  clinical diagnosis, 78, 79
  clinical features, 76
  course, 77
  definition, 75
  electrodiagnostic testing, 79
  epidemiology, 76
  laboratory testing, 79
  SDB, 87, 88
  symptoms
    dysphagia, 77
    leg weakness, 77
    localized muscle atrophy, 78
    muscle strength and exhaustibility
      measurement, 78
    myasthenic crisis, 78
    ocular symptoms, 77
    respiratory insufficiency, 78
    tongue weakness, 77

Myasthenia gravis (MG) (cont.)
   treatment
      AChEI, 79
      azathioprine, 80
      corticosteroids, 80
      cyclosporine A, 80
      intravenous immunoglobulin, 81
      mycophenolate mofetil, 81
      plasma exchange, 81
      tacrolimus (FK 506), 81
      thymectomy, 81
Myasthenic crisis (MC), 36, 38, 77, 78, 81
Myopathies and muscular dystrophies
   central hypersomnolence disorder, 66, 67
   circadian rhythm disorders, 67, 68
   insomnia, 64, 65
   parasomnias, 67
   SDB
      anatomical airway obstruction, 64
      coexisting cardiac abnormalities, 64
      diaphragmatic weakness, 63, 64
      lung volume reduction, 63
      normal breathing pattern, 62
      pathophysiological mechanism, 62, 63
      prevalence, 62
   sleep related movement disorders, 65, 66
Myotonic dystrophy (MD), 62, 64–67, 113

N
Nasal mask interface, 110
Negative-inspiratory force (NIF), 28, 31, 35, 37
Neurally adjusted ventilatory assist (NAVA), 120
Neuromechanical matching, 26, 38
Neuromuscular junction (NMJ)
   botulism (see Botulism)
   clinical features, 75
   definition, 73
   diagnosis of sleep issues, 89, 90
   LEMS (see Lambert–Eaton myasthenic syndrome (LEMS))
   treatment, 82
   motor end-plate with acetylcholine receptors, 74
   myasthenia gravis
      causes, 76
      clinical diagnosis, 78
      clinical features, 76
      course of, 77
      definition, 75
      electrodiagnostic testing, 79
      epidemiology, 75, 76
      laboratory testing, 79
      symptoms, 77, 78
      treatment, 79–81
   sleep disorders, 86, 87
   treatment, 90
Neuromuscular respiratory failure, 30
   causes, 26, 30
   evaluation, 26–28
   history and examinations, 31
   laboratory assessment, 28–30
   MV (see Mechanical ventilation (MV))
Nocturnal hypoventilation, 51, 96, 103, 104, 106, 108, 132
Nocturnal oximetry, 133
Nocturnal polysomnogram (NPSG), 15, 106
Nocturnal tests, 106–108
Non-invasive positive pressure ventilation (NIPPV), 108–110, 123, 125
Non-invasive ventilation (NIV)
   advantages, 118
   in ambulatory care, 124
   assisted coughing techniques, 135
   AVAPS, 124
   BIPAP, 36, 37, 109, 124
   BPAP, 133
   complications, 125–126, 135
   contraindications, 125–126, 134
   CPAP, 124, 133
   definition, 117, 122–123
   first-generation ventilators, 119
   fourth-generation ventilators, 120
   general principles, 119
   goals, 134
   indications, 124, 125
   initiation and management, 122, 123
   IPPV, 134
   NAVA, 120
   PEEP, 133
   physiological benefits, 117
   positive pressure ventilator, 120
   second-generation ventilators, 120
   SRBD, 108, 109
   third-generation ventilators, 120

O
Orbicularis oris weakness, 77
Obstructive sleep apnea (OSA), 9, 17, 50, 52, 62, 64, 84, 86, 87, 96, 97, 112, 121, 124, 139, 140, 142–144
Overlap syndrome, 51
Overnight oximetry, 107–108

P

Parasomnias, 67
Parasternal intercostals, 24
Pediatric NMD, 101
    diaphragmatic weakness, 102
    respiratory physiology, 102
    sleep-associated nocturnal respiratory disorders, 103
    SRBD (*see* Sleep-related breathing disorders (SRBD))
Pediatric polysomnography
    active sleep, 18
    indeterminate sleep, 18
    physiological variables, 17
    quiet sleep, 18
    respiratory scoring, 18
Periodic limb movements (PLMS), 7, 52, 89
Peripheral arterial tonometry (PAT)
    calibration, 11
    cost, 10
    measurement, 10
Peripheral neuropathy
    diaphragm palsy, 96
    MMNCB, 96
    restless legs syndrome, 97, 98
    risk factors, 96
    sleep apnea
        adult non-obese diabetics, 98
        CMT patients, 95
        compound muscle action potential, 96
        CPAP therapy, 97
        DPN, 98
        DSIS, 95
        sensory conduction velocity, 97
        severity, 96
        supramaximal stimulation, 97
    spinocerebellar ataxia, 97
Phrenic motor neurons, 25
Pittsburgh sleep quality index (PQSI), 90
Pneumography, 9
Polysomnogram study (PSG), 7, 10, 11, 17–18, 53, 55
Polysomnography, 5, 10, 11, 17, 97
    actigraphy, 16, 17
    airflow monitoring, 8, 9
    bi-level titration, 15
    body positioning and snoring, 9
    children (*see* Pediatric polysomnography)
    CPAP titration, 15
    definition, 1
    digital polygraphs, 3
    EEG (*see* Electroencephalography)
    EKG, 8
    EMG, 7, 8
    end-tidal CO_2, 15
    EOG, 8
    evolution, 1, 2
    gastroesophageal studies, 10
    HST, 17
    indications, 10
    MSLT, 16
    MWT, 16
    NPSG, 15
    PAT
        calibration, 11
        cost, 10
        montage (*see* Montage)
    RBD, 16
    sleep laboratory/sleep center, 4
    sleep staging and scoring, 2, 3
    split study, 15
    SRBD, 106–107
    technical considerations, 3, 4
Positive airway pressure (PAP) therapy
    battery-powered PAP machines, 148
    claustrophobia, 143
    contour PAP pillows, 148
    device maintenance, 148
    during travel, 148
    education, 140
    gel/rubber cushion, 143
    humidification problems, 146–148
    machines, 140
    mask air-leak, 144
    mask interface, 143
    mask pressure, 144–145
    mouth air-leak, 144
    noise level, 145–146
    patient compliance, 149
    patient day-to-day challenges, 140
    pressure intolerance, 141, 142
    sleep apnea, 139, 140
    symptoms, 149
    tubing problem, 146
Positive end expiratory pressure (PEEP), 121
Positive occipital sharp transients (POSTS), 6
Positive pressure ventilator, 120
Posterior dominant rhythm/posterior alpha rhythm, 5
Posterior slow waves of youth, 7
Pre-Botzinger complex, 25, 38
Primary lateral sclerosis (PLS), 48
Progressive muscular atrophy (PMA), *see* Sporadic Lower motor neuron syndromes
Pseudoperiodic lateralized epileptiform discharges (PLEDs), 7

R

Rapid eye movement (REM) sleep, 96
Rapid repetitive nerve stimulation (RNS), 86
REM behavior disorder (RBD), 16
REM sleep without atonia (RSWA), 52, 67
Renshaw cells, 25
Resistance to ischemic conduction block (RICB), 97
Respiratory effort related arousals (RERAs), 8, 17
Respiratory failure
  diagnosis, 132
  laboratory assessment, 28 (*see* Neuromuscular respiratory failure)
  NMD classification, 130, 131
  pathophysiology, 131, 132
  symptoms, 133
Respiratory function, neurophysiology, 130
Respiratory inductive plethysmography (RIP), 9
Respiratory magnetometers, 9
Respiratory muscles
  expiratory muscles, 24, 25
  inspiratory muscles, 23, 24
Restless legs syndrome (RLS), 52, 65, 66, 87–89, 97, 98
Retrotrapezoid nucleus/parafacial respiratory group (RTN/pFRG), 25
Riluzole, 48
R-K scoring system, 5
Rostral ventral respiratory group (rVRG), 25

S

Scalene muscles, 24
Scapuloperoneal SMA (SPSMA), 46
Second-generation ventilators, 119–120
Seronegative MG, 76, 79
Single-breath test, 90
Sleep disordered breathing (SDB)
  central sleep apnea, 52
  mixed sleep apnea, 52
  nocturnal hypoventilation, 51
  obstructive sleep apnea, 51
Sleep fragmentation, 51
Sleep onset REM periods (SOREMPs, 67
Sleep-associated nocturnal respiratory disorders, 103
Sleep-Disordered Breathing in Neuromuscular Disease Questionnaire (SINQ-5), 89
Sleep-related breathing disorders (SRBD), 112
  adverse clinical effects, 110
  assessment, 105
  clinical history, 104, 105
  definition, 101
  diagnostic and clinical evaluation, 104

diurnal tests, 105, 106
HMV, 111
invasive mechanical ventilation, 109, 110
nasal mask interface, 110
NIPPV, 108, 109
overnight oximetry, 107, 108
polysomnography, 106–107
predictors, 105
prevalence, 101
sleep-related central hypoventilation, 103
symptoms, 103
SMA, *see* Spinal muscular atrophy (SMA)
Small sharp spikes (SSS), 7
Sniff nasal inspiratory pressure (SNIP), 54
Spinal and bulbar muscular atrophy (X-Linked), 46
Spinal muscular atrophy (SMA), 112, 113
  clinical features, 44
  incidence, 44
  Kennedy's disease, 46
  LOSMoN, 46
  SMA-LED, 46
  SPSMA, 46
  type 0, 45
  type 1, 45
  type 2, 45
  type 3, 45
  type 4, 45
Spinocerebellar ataxia (SCA), 97
SPSMA, *see* Scapuloperoneal SMA (SPSMA)
Strain gauges, 9

T

TENSILON test, 79
Thermistors, 9
Thermocouples, 9
Third-generation ventilators, 120
Thymomas, 76
Thymus gland, 76
Tracheostomy ventilation, 135
Transdiaphragmatic pressure (Pdi), 29

V

Vertex sharp waves, 7
Vital capacity, 27, 28, 32, 35, 36, 38, 39

W

WatchPAT system, 10
Wicket rhythms, 7
Willis Ekbom disease, 88, 89
Willis-Ekbom disease, *see* Restless legs syndrome (RLS)

The manufacturer's authorised representative in the EU is Springer Nature Customer Service Centre GmbH, Europaplatz 3, 69115 Heidelberg, Germany. If you have any concerns regarding our products, please contact ProductSafety@springernature.com

Printed and bound by CPI Group (UK) Ltd, Croydon, CR0 4YY

23/03/2026

02076369-0009